CHOLERA

CHOLERA

The Biography

Christopher Hamlin

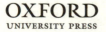
OXFORD
UNIVERSITY PRESS

OXFORD
UNIVERSITY PRESS

Great Clarendon Street, Oxford OX2 6DP

Oxford University Press is a department of the University of Oxford.
It furthers the University's objective of excellence in research, scholarship,
and education by publishing worldwide in

Oxford New York

Auckland Cape Town Dar es Salaam Hong Kong Karachi
Kuala Lumpur Madrid Melbourne Mexico City Nairobi
New Delhi Shanghai Taipei Toronto

With offices in

Argentina Austria Brazil Chile Czech Republic France Greece
Guatemala Hungary Italy Japan Poland Portugal Singapore
South Korea Switzerland Thailand Turkey Ukraine Vietnam

Oxford is a registered trade mark of Oxford University Press
in the UK and in certain other countries

Published in the United States
by Oxford University Press Inc., New York

British Library Cataloguing in Publication Data
Data available

Library of Congress Cataloging-in-Publication Data
Hamlin, Christopher, 1951–
Cholera : the biography / Christopher Hamlin.
p. ; cm.—(Biographies of disease)
Includes bibliographical references and index.
ISBN 978-0-19-954624-4 (hardback : alk. paper)
1. Cholera—History—19th century. 2. Cholera—History—20th century.
I. Title. II. Series: Biographies of disease (Oxford, England)
[DNLM: 1. Cholera—history. 2. History, 19th Century.
3. History, 20th Century. WC 262 H223c 2009]
RA644.C3H28 2009
614.5'14—dc22 2009026414

Typeset by SPI Publisher Services, Pondicherry, India
Printed in Great Britain
on acid-free paper by Clays Ltd, St Ives plc

ISBN 978-0-19-954624-4

1 3 5 7 9 10 8 6 4 2

ACKNOWLEDGEMENTS

The author thanks Jessica Weaver and Angharad, Fern, and Kat Hamlin for research and editing help, and Bill and Helen Bynum for their judicious mix of encouragement and critique.

I would like to express my great debt and thanks to the many historians and other cholera scholars whose studies I have drawn on. In a more academic work these pages would be thick with specific references to their works. Citation conventions of this series minimize use of notes in favor of a "Further Reading" section where those works are cited and situated. But if the specific references are rare, the debt is no less deep; a great joy of this project has been the privilege of engaging with the rich and insightful scholarship on cholera.

CONTENTS

LIST OF ILLUSTRATIONS

PROLOGUE: HOME ALONE

"'I am Mary Lennox,' the little girl said, drawing herself up stiffly… 'I fell asleep when everyone had the cholera and I have only just wakened up. Why does nobody come?'" No one comes because most are dead. Nine-year old Mary's query in some unnamed south Asian cantonment in 1906 opens Frances Hodgson Burnett's *The Secret Garden* (1911). The spoiled child is vexed that her personal servant has not come— her "Ayah" has not only taken the cholera but had the audacity to die of it. So, too, have her mother and father. The servants had died or fled; "the people were dying like flies." Cholera produced panic; "noise and hurrying about and wailing" frighten Mary. Social order breaks down: "when people had the cholera it seemed that they remembered nothing but themselves." But cholera would also lead (as it does for Mary at Mistlethwaite Manor in North Yorkshire) to soul searching and sometimes to remarkable altruism.

Most of us need not fear cholera zapping our parents overnight. Yet cholera still terrifies. Mostly it is in abeyance. It constitutes only a small fraction of global diarrhea. But it is feared for its relentless ability to spread, its suddenness, and its deadliness.

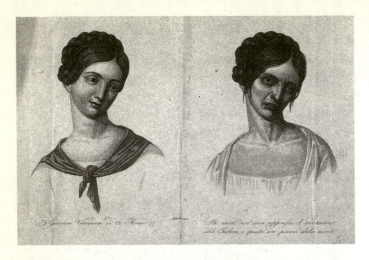

1. The cholera was known as the 'blue' disease. Dehydration caused a sunken, cadaverous countenance and changed the hue of the skin (*Wellcome Library, London*)

The term, if not the experience, resonates. Cholera *struck*: the term is especially apposite. It could be anticipated, for its pandemics approached slowly. For most of the nineteenth century it could not reliably be prevented, avoided, or cured. For most of the twentieth, it could be (and was often) avoided; it could be (but was not always) prevented or cured. But what it did, it can do again.

Cholera did not merely kill, and rapidly, but it distorted lives and bodies. It took hold, drawing out the body's heat, twisting muscles into spasms and cramps, producing insatiable thirst but taking away voice. It liquefied a body as fluids streamed uncontrollably and insensibly from both ends. It quickly wrung the water from the body, leaving a shriveled form and thickened blood. All this in a few hours. Cholera bypassed both the cathartic crisis of fever and the advances and declines of consumption; it was not a disease that a person lived with.

Cholera was experienced not simply by its victims but by their communities, both immediate and broader, and not only *during* epidemics but before and after them. It was an ordeal of anticipation, for much of cholera's story is a story of fear. My own referent is three decades of contemplating nuclear annihilation: much time spent hoping to hope, yet anticipating a disaster that would not only kill, but destroy both material and communal bases of society, uproot faith in any cosmic order. Massive nuclear war has not yet come; cholera did, repeatedly.

The nature of the beast

How many died? Figures abound, but rarely do we know much about how they were arrived at. Often numbers of cholera deaths were not mere facts, but attempts to shock—or to deny. Some are wild guesses, some are lies. Only a few have gone beyond claims by checking graves dug or coffin costs. The records for India (and Pakistan) for 1877–1954 represent a reasonable degree of institutional continuity in a part of the world where cholera was endemic. There were 22 million deaths, with decadal cholera mortality rising as high as 1.5/1,000 in 1887–96, equivalent to 429,000 average annual cholera deaths.[1] But elsewhere averages mislead, for cholera was a rare visitor and by no means the greatest killer of the nineteenth century. When it came, it was quick, often deadly to those stricken, but a place might be hit heavily or lightly. And even if we knew who was counting and how, we might still be confused: modern clinicians not only find cholera hard to distinguish from other severe diarrhea; they also disagree as to how it should be defined.

3

Along with its deadliness, cholera's relentless spreading was a key feature. Over the course of the nineteenth century it appeared in almost every corner of the world, and in many places repeatedly. By mid century most perceived a pattern of recurrent waves, moving outward from India, the first beginning in 1817, each dying out after 15–30 years, soon to be followed by the next. All but the seventh, which began in Sulawesi, came from Bengal; many traced the same routes to the northwest, equally to the southeast. If the larger picture of pandemics seemed clear, details of itinerary, even chronology, were not. Analysts did not agree on the bounding of pandemics. The most common list has seven: 1817–24 (1st), 1829–51 (2nd) (listed by some as three semi-distinct pandemics), 1852–9 (3rd), 1860–75 (4th), 1881–95 (5th), 1899–1923 (6th), 1960– (7th).[2]

It is in the magnitude of the *reaction* to it that cholera stands out as the signal disease of the nineteenth century. It was (apparently) new as an epidemic entity and grew up in conjunction with Enlightenment liberalism, nationalism, imperialism, and the rise of global biomedical science. It was most problematic— as opposed to causing the greatest mortality—in precisely the places where these darlings thrived. It looms large in British history, though Britain was hit lightly and rarely. Seen in terms of the evolving social contract between rich and poor, it was not just a deadly event but a violation of emerging expectations.

Cholera's greatest insult was to progress itself. Not as a disease that individuals died from but as an invader of continent, state, or town, cholera violated a sense of a European identity that was being applied to other places as they succumbed to civilization. Ever-spreading death might be allowed for the benighted past, and temporarily acknowledged as the unfortunate condition of the present benighted, but it was not permissible in these happy days of science—both of physical science and of *Staatswissenschaft*.

In places where there was a faith in progress, cholera was someone's fault, something to be fixed. But who was letting in the rough beast, and how? Cholera raised questions of the accountability of states (even more acutely as they came to see themselves as nation states) to their people(s). Those people might be citizens, or subjects, or indigenes who happened to occupy a valuable colony. Obligations to these groups varied. As Mary's narrative hints, the obliteration of large numbers of "natives" might not be problematic except insofar as it involved transmission of a deadly disease to those who mattered more.

Cholera also raised problems of accountability to a liberal world order. Progress was to be a product of liberty. Free and safe movement of ideas and goods, but equally free use of property and capital, were to bring progress. These were matters of right as well as of good. But often it seemed that these rights could be delivered only by being denied, for fear of cholera brought about a regime of international surveillance, coercion, even confinement in what can best be called concentration camps, like those for the quarantine of Muslim pilgrims, to whom freedom of movement was not a liberal value but a mode of religious expression (and, therefore, dispensable). Domestically too, cholera led to a regime in which civil rights—to face the disease in one's home, hold on to one's clothes and bedclothes, follow ordinary hygienic habits, practice funerary customs—might be suspended or transformed for the common good. We may view curtailment as sometimes justified; in other cases as reflecting the unanswerable force of fear. But in either case, such authoritarianism did not mesh well with liberal values. Surely, the intercourse of free persons could not be the spreading of death? That nature should exact biological demands inconsistent with its moral and economic instructions was hard to accept.

Coercion was no substitute for cooperation; and accountability came to rest with individual persons. For it turned out that whatever policies a state might make, stopping cholera required the cooperation of everyone. Thus, the states that were to be accountable to their citizens deflected responsibility back onto those citizens, making them accountable to it. Baffled by the happenstance of cholera, doctors would often attribute it to the failing of an individual. A single hygienic error, even insufficient cheeriness of mind, might bring on an outbreak. Cholera had to be handled at the most intimate levels of civil society—in village or neighborhood. It preferentially struck the marginalized, and was both a mark of marginality and an incentive to assimilate or reassimilate the marginalized. Hence cholera, in exhibiting interdependence, helped transform subjects and indigenes into at least a kind of citizen: the property to kill others with one's excretions, is after all, a kind of property.

And what pertained at these intimate levels of civil society carried over to the grander level too. For the microbe in the bowels of the single person might introduce cholera not only to a village, but, as was repeatedly the case, to a continent. More than any other infectious disease, cholera brought the world together. The fate of all might be in the bowels of any. Or such, we can safely say, was the lesson learned in the long run. But it was (and is) often resisted. The prospect of cholera often led to the heightening of racial and class distinctions and tensions.

Behind all these was capitalism. Cholera coincided with its rise; one may even say that cholera was a problem of capitalism. They intersected in many ways. The "dark satanic mills," the Coketowns of the Industrial Revolution in England and elsewhere, are paradigmatic sites of cholera epidemics. Yet cholera was rural as well as urban, and more heavily associated with port or market than with industrial town. More important is the premium on the movement of peoples and goods, and the national and international structures that maintained trade. The problem of cholera, as the American Edward Shakespeare would make clear, was of making the world safe for commerce. But to many, concentrated capital was also the solution: grand investments in infrastructure organized people into, ideally, cholera-free piped cities.

The response to cholera indeed reflects paradoxes associated with capitalism. A global problem required parochial responses. Fatalism coexisted with the presumption of control; atomistic individualism with communitarianism. An event that in its inevitability seemed beyond meaning, and simply natural, became laden with meaning. The great need for regulation exhibited the ultimate impotence of regulators—still the case today. In our security-conscious world of passports and bureaucracies, it is often smugglers who pass on cholera.[3] Marx would smile.

Cholera evolving

Cholera also grew up as a subject of rapidly changing biomedical science. At the beginning of the nineteenth century the term referred to a generic constitutional condition. It would become a specific invasive disease well before there was any clear concept of an invasive agent. By late in the century cholera had become the exemplar of the new germ theory, which, by defining the disease in terms of its microbe, transformed cholera epidemiology. For most of the twentieth century cholera was a laboratory science. When truths of laboratory and of field clashed, as they did regularly in the development of cholera vaccines, laboratory usually prevailed—reduction and simplification would ultimately make sense of it all. It was not until around 1960, as the seventh pandemic began to spread, that a more productive reciprocity between field and laboratory began to arise, one based on a fruitful interplay of disciplines ranging from molecular genetics to ecology. It brought (and brings) great insight into the disease, but neither reduction nor simplicity. Questions that had been pushed aside—like the periodicity of pandemics or the variable character of the disease—suddenly seemed important again.

A perusal of bibliographies is a good way to trace the evolution of "cholera." For the heyday of cholera, the four series of the *Index-Catalogue of the Surgeon-General's Library* (1882, 1898, 1922, and 1938) are revealing. During the nineteenth century cholera was the chief site of a centuries-old debate about whether epidemics were to be attributed to the spread of some specific contagious substance or to a local or global environmental shift. The phenomena of cholera were ambiguous, and the rival positions often misconceived, but the expenditure of ink was enormous. Great attention was given to assembling the history and statistics of cholera in the hope that the circumstances of each outbreak would ultimately gestate into general laws by which cholera might be managed.

By the 1898 edition, bacteriology had taken over. If Robert Koch was not the first to see the cholera microbe, his isolation in 1883–4 of what is now called *Vibrio cholerae* was a watershed. A new heading for "inoculation" had appeared. By the first quarter of the twentieth century cholera has lost its "Asiatic" modifier, just as it was becoming almost exclusively (if temporarily) Asian. The final two series reflect the shift from epidemic and clinic to laboratory. There is a heading for "experimental" cholera, and the "Cholera Vibrio" gets equal billing with "Cholera" itself.

Since the mid 1950s, historians of many sorts have focused on cholera. Biomedical scientists began to mine the cholera legacy for object lessons in the late 1930s. The disease seemed to have receded into the Asian mists, and its "conquest" elsewhere could be celebrated. It is at this time that the famous, if often mistold, story of the anesthesiologist-epidemiologist John Snow (1813–58) and the Broad Street pump becomes familiar as an exemplar of epidemiological method. There was similar enthusiasm for the Prussian bacteriologist Robert Koch (1843–1910), even though his observation and isolation of the agent of cholera in Egypt and Calcutta in 1883–4 could not immediately be confirmed by his eponymous "postulates," the experimental protocol for demonstrating a cause-and-effect relationship between putative agent and disease.

Two others often enter into such accounts. One is the Florentine Filipo Pacini (1812–83), after whom *Vibrio cholerae* is named. Pacini observed the microbe in the mid 1850s (others may have too), but, more importantly, he developed over a decade a comprehensive, quantitative, and largely accurate description of cholera pathology. But Florence was not the center of science it had been in Galileo's day, and Pacini's papers were passed over. The moral has been less "send to the best journals" than "virtue may have to be its own reward for a long time but sooner or later credit will get to the right place."[4] If Pacini's is an ambivalent tale, then that of Max von Pettenkofer (1818–1901) is classic tragedy: "pride goeth before the fall." In the days before Koch, Pettenkofer, Professor of Hygiene at Munich, ruled European cholera science with a mix of obscure theory and meaningless data. He would not admit that progress lay in bacteriology and in his younger colleague Koch. Defiant, he and his disciples swallowed cultures of the supposed cholera agent. They lived on, unrepentant, though Pettenkofer, as befits the tragedy in which he was principal, shot himself in 1901.

Plainly there were giants in those days. By comparison, the others who wrote the innumerable tracts and treatises on cholera are largely anonymous—boors and fools, purveyors of bizarre therapies who serve for comic relief in older histories of medicine, and together serve as the backdrop of dull stupidity against which the work of the heroes shines forth the more brilliantly.

Cholera was slower to come under the gaze of professional historians. When it did, these were by no means primarily medical historians. In the 1960s cholera arose as a social historian's probe, as a part of efforts to explain class politics in the industrializing world. For Louis Chevalier (1958), Roderick McGrew (1960), Asa Briggs (1961), and Charles Rosenberg (1962, 1966), cholera epidemics let us in to "see society."[5] Epidemics brought down officials who poked their noses into slums and filled reports with observations and summations. Their counting and describing meant that cholera provided "a unique opportunity to penetrate class structure, social attitudes, and the living conditions of a broad segment of the population."[6] Even better, cholera returned periodically. One could use successive cholera epidemics to calibrate cultural change, as did Rosenberg, who made the first three American epidemics (in 1832, 1848–54, and 1866) an instrument to chart changes in Americans' notions of God's government of the world and individual and social sin and responsibility. Cholera was "a *natural sampling device* for the social historian."[7]

But cholera was no mere occasion for an open house. Observation was tied up with intervention. As well as a way to see what had been hidden, cholera was a way to gauge social forces that could not otherwise be measured. Cholera crises ripped aside ideology to reveal social reality. As McGrew, following Chevalier, put it: "Epidemics, and perhaps other major calamities, do not create abnormal situations, rather they emphasize normal aspects of abnormal situations...An epidemic intensifies certain behavior patterns, but those patterns, instead of being aberrations, betray deeply rooted and continuing social imbalances."[8] Why things were most real when most raw was never quite clear.

The context of this work was Marxist. A revolutionary consummation of industrial society was the default of social development. As exacting tests of societal strength, cholera epidemics might be seen—most clearly for Chevalier—as potentially revolution-precipitating events. Especially for France, the apparent coincidence of cholera with uprisings (in 1832 and 1848) and, more broadly, the common phenomenon of inter-class cholera riots confirmed that potential.

That cholera did not precipitate revolution was seen to demonstrate an underappreciated degree of stability, most evident in the sanitary and social-reform movements of the nineteenth century. Cholera triggered investigations; investigations led to recognition of the effects of insanitation and squalor; reform of social conditions dulled the edge of the unacceptability of proletarian existence, allowing gradual expansion of the franchise in conjunction with the maintenance of social order (even on an international scale) and the flourishing of capitalism. Cholera is still often seen as a friend to "reform."

Could a model so plausible not be true? One often still encounters in the modern public-health literature a faith that a good cholera will cut through hygienic apathy and make the money flow. But historians were finding their own idea too pat. The coincidence of cholera with social unrest proved misleading. Rioters were pressing immediate and local issues, not class concerns. Inquiry-based reform was time-consuming, costly, and contentious; often governments deployed old plague measures while pretending that these were grounded in the best modern science. Cholera might provide an occasion for sanitary reform, but its quickly passing outbreaks rarely sufficed for long-term planning and institutional change. For political radicals it was a distraction. Snow's proof that cholera spread in water has not brought good water to all, however much it should have done. Improving water supplies was propelled by industry and demand for middle-class amenity more than by disease prevention.

As bearers of polity, nation states might be the right units for revolution or reform, but they were generally not the main site of cholera response. What could be done was done locally. Finely grained urban studies explored both the dynamics of cholera response and its variability: families and neighborhoods; insiders and outsiders; particular landowners, employers, or magistrates; local customs and modes of making a living; all had a great deal to do both with cholera's impact and with the response to it.

Colonial cholera was a partial exception. The trappings of autocracy might be more visible in colonies, but there too they were distributed and diluted. Not town councils, but quasi-military districts or great estates were apt to be the units of response. Far from igniting revolution or stimulating reform, colonial cholera more often reinforced racism. Revulsion toward the poor had been part of European cholera conversation, but there reform could be done at arm's length, looking away and holding one's nose. The dangerous and disgusting classes of Paris or London might be emasculated by the water and sewers of civilization. In South Asia, the problems seemed of another magnitude. There, evidently, people lived and died by different rules. Apparently, they had different expectations and therefore different needs; that cholera had supposedly always been there explained their supposed apathy toward its prevention. The inertia bound up in that cycle of poverty and disease was too vast to oppose; one could hope only to divert it from the cantonments in which little Mary Lennox and her parents had holed up.

With the fading of Marxism, interest in imagined communities made of words displaced interest in things. Even class, the social historian's holdfast, was borne off, transformed from hours, wages, and prices into shared language. Vanishing too was the hope that a simple and single story could be told. The first social histories of cholera had been carried out in a golden age, when the maturation of history into a rigorous social science seemed possible (and near). Truly comparative studies using "cholera" as a "tool," whether of illumination, analysis, or even transformation, required seeing "cholera" as a single well-defined entity: it was vital (and therefore possible) to distinguish nature from culture, cholera ideology from cholera science.

But in learning to see colonial cholera through the eyes of European or American officials, historians, ironically, ran the risk of losing sight of the disease in highlighting its representation, just as their sources had done. Their relentless deployment of images of dirt, disgust, and deadly danger had made cholera less a disease in real persons and more a representation of horror. Their language was both powerful and historically important—it illustrated the pervasive institutions of discipline identified by Michel Foucault; it was a field for the subtle linguistic microphysics by which chaos could be made into order, or the disparate behaviors of individuals could be forged into a "social body." Cholera too went through a linguistic turn; a recent monograph on cholera, Gilbert's *Cholera and Nation* (2008), is a contribution to English literature and is not isolated or idiosyncratic in that field.

"Cholera" was and is literary; what we have made that word mean dictates what we have done and what we do about diseases that are its referent. But, just as cholera is more than a microbe—a Gram negative, facultative anaerobe—it is also more than "cholera-talk."

Mostly, cholera histories have been about something else—scientific method and the conduct of scientists, social experience, the relations of governments to peoples, racism and injustice, and the power of words. *All these approaches* help to make sense of the composite cholera that each author presumes and seeks to enlist. And yet we miss an important whole. "Cholera" as class relations is a drawing-room farce of mistaken identity. The framework may be plain, but we miss fear, bewilderment, uncertainty, desperation, and, for that matter, diarrhea. Equally, the bacteriologist's or epidemiologist's cholera is often narrow and rigid, a show trial that vindicates the present at the expense of oversimplifying the past and condemning most of its inhabitants to stupidity, inhumanity, even venality.

So what would cholera's own story be?

Cholera's story would not be simply the natural history of a microbe, the pathological history of human bodies it infests, or even the distribution of such bodies in time and space. It would include experiments and therapies; hospitals, gallons of disinfectant, water filters, and border guards; rectal swabs and culture plates; tracts and sermons; peer-refereed journal articles and grant applications; unnumbered meetings and careers; also acute suffering and death of millions of lonely persons, and equally their fear, and sometimes their relief.

I wrote earlier of cholera as "presumed" and "enlisted." Cholera has often been treated as a unitary and unchanging entity, and also as a dead and well-anatomized thing. Around 1960 when the cholera history projects began, most saw cholera as essentially over. Its microbe agent and that agent's means of transmission had long been known. It could be cured. It lingered in corners of Asia; if you were going there you got a shot. Hence the great comprehensive cholera treatise of R. Pollitzer, prepared for the World Health Organization in the mid 1950s, reads as a case-closing summary. There are loose ends, but an authority undertakes to digest such a mass of knowledge only on the assumption that it will not have to be done again. In any case, most historians had already stopped with Koch, who, it seemed, had answered all the big questions.

We used cholera as a tool of historical or literary insight because we assumed it to be fixed, to be beyond history and to lie outside words. Seemingly under control in the larger world, it figured easily in our narratives, a simple noun available to occasion public crisis. The exception was the French historian François Delaporte. Recognizing that the term and concept of cholera had entered Paris in 1832 at a time of tense class relations, Delaporte studied the deployment of the term, without claiming to know anything about the biological states it presumably referred to. Since those he studied had no access to the entity articulated by Snow, Koch, and their successors, Delaporte's historian had no business interpreting their actions in terms of such an entity. Such agnosticism permitted a standpoint of equality to rival persons and institutions in their efforts to command the term "cholera."

Was Delaporte right? He did manage to present cholera as open, not fixed. Yet he neglected much. If he was right to read "cholera" as sign not thing, he left out the lived experience. He was also ambivalent toward the frameworks, the intellectual and institutional contexts, by which signs gained meaning, and conviction led to practice.

Delaporte's picture of cholera in Paris in 1832, of flux in its many forms, fits cholera post-Pollitzer remarkably well. Even as Pollitzer wrote, the pathology of cholera was being elucidated through isolation of a toxin that disrupted osmotic balance. The seventh pandemic (caused by a different *Vibrio cholerae* biotype) would soon start; conventions about the stability of the microbe, its pathology, transmission, and control would be overturned in the next half century, in many cases repeatedly. Formerly Asian, cholera became prominent in Latin America and Africa.

Despite vast investment in its study, the answer to the simple question "what is this cholera?" remains elusive. No longer is it possible to claim with confidence to *know* cholera. With cholera changing and inchoate, the control in our social and historical experiments has vanished. What had seemed most solid about it, its microbe, has turned out (like other microbes) to be a repository for varying bits of rogue DNA, which together express toxicity under certain conditions. While we know vastly more about it, the general entity "cholera" is less fixed than at any time since 1830.

But we should not need the current flux in cholera science and cholera incidence to convince us that cholera writ large is a work in progress—that it is not just an evolving organism but a composite of ideology, political structures, class relations, systems of food, water, and sanitation, of learned knowledge (even in disciplines far beyond the biomedical sciences), and even of changing environment and climate. That composite is more than an occasion for surveillance or a stimulus for reforms that are bound to happen. It is an evolving historical agent in its own right, folding in its own past, but belonging to the spheres of creativity and contingency. We have no business pinning it down, but are hard pressed to keep up. This cholera was at the vanguard of many modes of biomedical science and practice. Cholera was the first focus of modern biomedical diplomacy: the International Sanitary Conferences, beginning in 1851, which would work out uniform standards to minimize disease transmission, were for the rest of the century concerned almost exclusively with cholera. It has been and is the locus of trenchant social criticism. A disease among the poor, it has seemed to indicate societal failure.

Seeing cholera—composite cholera—as agent, brings us to biography. Cholera has long been personified, but only to demonize. Seeking to be Boswell to its Johnson, I shall continue to personify. Chapter 1, treating the period leading up to the first pandemic, considers cholera as idea, first as a component of the humoral pathology, then as a scourge of the timeless East. There I explore how it became so closely associated with India. Chapter 2 focuses on the second and third pandemics (1829–60), and has cholera gaining an identity, or "finding itself." The primary concern there is with the cultural response to cholera. Chapter 3 takes the story into the 1880s, the fifth pandemic, and is concerned with cholera's political status and incorporation into administrative structures, as "Citizen Cholera." Chapters 4 and 5 address the comprehension of cholera—cholera science. Here cholera is a subject on an analyst's couch, baffling before 1884; thereafter confined in laboratories, to be reduced to ever more ultimate entities: serotypes, genes, proteins and polymers. Chapter 6, "Cholera's last laugh," brings us to the present. It reflects on the Latin American epidemic of the 1990s, the early twenty-first century outbreaks among refugees, but also the new ecological view of cholera microbiology. There cholera breaks free—equally as pathogenic microbe and as scientific concept.

I

CHOLERA: THE VERY IDEA

For years, when someone in our family got the "runs," we referred to it as having cholera—thankful that it was not the real thing.

For most in the modern world that real thing is a disease resulting from infection by the cholera microbe (up to 1993, *Vibrio cholerae* O1, in either its "classical" or its "El Tor" biotype). That deadly and spreading disease had begun to push northwest and southeast from Bengal in 1817 and has, most believe, spread from that nucleus repeatedly. Yet, as a term, "cholera" had been around long before. It fulfilled a categorical imperative in the ancient Hippocratic scheme of the four humors: health was a balance of blood, phlegm, black bile, and yellow bile, individualized in terms of one's temperament. The expulsion of excess yellow bile (*choler*) was, when severe enough to constitute an illness, a cholera (*morbus*). In the early nineteenth century, when Europeans spoke of having cholera, they usually meant gastroenteritis with vomiting *and* diarrhea, which was presumed to accomplish that expulsion. That was what we meant by cholera; it was the "cholera" that Samuel Taylor Coleridge had in 1804, and that suffered by Captain Charles Frankland RN traveling in the Near East in the late 1820s.

> This morning early, I was disagreeably surprised by a violent attack of diarrhoea (cholera morbus), accompanied by vomiting, which confined me all the day to my bed. I knew how to treat this malady, from former experience in South America, and did nothing but fast and drink syrup of orjeat and water. Mr Parish, attached to the embassy, was so good as to...send for the physician...but ere the healer came, the violence of the malady was over; and he told me that I could do nothing better than follow up mine own prescription.

As in Frankland's case, it was not usually a severe disease, nor a spreading one.

That shift in the years after 1817, from cholera as a transitory state of one's constitution to cholera as a relentless and deadly invader, was neither quick nor unproblematic. At first, the similarities had seemed clear enough to warrant using the old term. After 1830, "cholera" (or spasmodic, epidemic, or later "Asiatic" cholera) would refer to the new pandemic disease, leaving *cholera morbus* or *cholera nostras* ("our cholera," as opposed to a foreign import), for the old disease. Even then the distinction was not clear cut. A series of terms—"cholerine," "choleroid," "choleraic diarrhea," or "paracholera"—would be coined for transitional forms.

For, then and now, it was by no means obvious how to distinguish the old friendly diarrhea from the new invading enemy. Usually, one distinguished by context, and retrospectively. The most important criteria have been severity and epidemicity. The new "cholera" was highly fatal, the old usually self-limiting. The old cholera occasionally struck an isolated town, but did not spread from continent to continent. But these were judgment calls, impossible to make at the beginning of what *might be* an epidemic, when it was not clear how many would be stricken or how severely.

By about 1900, the old cholera was no longer a real disease (except perhaps in the households of historians of medicine). The transitional labels were gone by about 1960. "Cholera," however severe, had come to be defined by its agent. Illnesses that had once warranted that label went on the scrap heap of generic gastroenteritis caused by other microbes or none. For most practical purposes, the new, "true," cholera could be put there too. Most of these severe diarrhoeas could be prevented by disrupting fecal–oral transfer and cured by oral rehydration.

Often, in tracing cholera's history, we have wanted to focus on the "real thing," on disease, not name. The older "cholera" is simply a distraction when we ask questions like "had this new disease existed earlier, in India or elsewhere?" It is a question we cannot answer. Paleopathology does not help; reliance on descriptions of symptoms is treacherous. Gastroenteritis leading to collapse can have many causes. To expect each language to have a term for the precise clinical entity we call cholera is absurd: one need only reflect how much cholera's meaning has changed in European languages in two centuries. People group symptoms and explain pathologies differently. Meanings evolve. "Cholera" was, to some, part of a continuum involving diarrhea and dysentery; to others, a bilious colic. More important than "what did they call cholera?" is "what is gained and lost in these meaning changes"? For we have no business simply presiding over the theft of the old cholera's identity in the name of the manifest destiny of biomedical science. That translation of cholera—from ours and everyone's to the Asians'—had profound consequences for relations between nations and between peoples. The vision of "cholera" as a scourge from the dirty parts of the world to the clean still affects efforts to deal with the larger problem of global diarrheal disease.

A "perfect cholera"

Like a cold that may have many symptoms, cholera was a concept before it was a disease.[1] It could appear in various degrees of perfection.

Pull works from the shelves of a late-eighteenth-century medical library: there will be mention, usually brief, of cholera in texts on practice. It was also dealt with in most family medical guides and in works of medical geography. But few publications were on cholera alone; it was not a disease of learned interest or a research frontier. Cholera was neither particularly common nor problematic. In the 785 cases treated in 1783 in the Carlisle Dispensary, there were three of *cholera morbus*, along with 40 of "looseness," and 66 of "stomach complaints."[2] As this list hints, the learned term coexisted with other lay and professional designations. In England the physician's "cholera" might have been the lay person's "griping of the guts," while in France not only was there *la grippe*, but also *trousse gallant*.[3] Usually, the symptom that warranted "cholera" rather than a generic belly aching was the combination of continued diarrhea and vomiting, together with spasms and cramps in the limbs.

Good accounts of its course, causes, and therapies were often still drawn from Aretaeus of Cappadocia (*c.* CE 50) and the North African Caelius Aurelianus (probably fifth century CE). Both were sources for the long entry on cholera in Robert James's three volume *Medicinal Dictionary* (1743–5). James (1703–76), founder of a famous proprietary fever powder, was a friend of Dr Samuel Johnson; the two advised on each other's dictionaries. Here James relies on moderns too: his work is effectively a review article on all aspects of cholera and my main source here.

Within humoral medicine, cholera was not necessarily a disease. Periodically, a body might need to expel excess bile as a health-restoring act. Bile was "natural clyster," noted the late-seventeenth-century Danish physician Caspar Bartholin. Generally, that expulsion came in the summer or early autumn and was seen as a seasonal readjustment. *Cholera morbus* simply suggested an unusual degree of this normal occurrence. As "choleric" reminds us, biliousness was also associated with "a fierce and Wrathful Disposition." That already linked cholera with the tropics, where barbarity reigned and disease was more intense, and with hot and sultry tropical weather that could visit temperate latitudes.

By James's time, cholera had broadened from its classical humoral origins. It still usually involved the expulsion of bile; quite why or how was less clear. The Hippocratic writers had conceived two kinds: the dry cholera—of eructation and flatulence—and a moist cholera of vomiting and diarrhea. But Bossier de Sauvages in the mid eighteenth century identified eleven. The so-called *cholera sicca* (not, probably, the same as the Hippocratic dry cholera) complicated matters. It brought neither vomiting nor diarrhea, just quick collapse and death, and would come to be viewed as the deadliest form of cholera. Its key symptom was the intense coldness of the limbs.

That breadth was reflected in a wide range of views as to which symptoms were primary and which incidental. It was not obvious that cholera was a species of diarrhea, even if controlling diarrhea might be important in managing the disease.

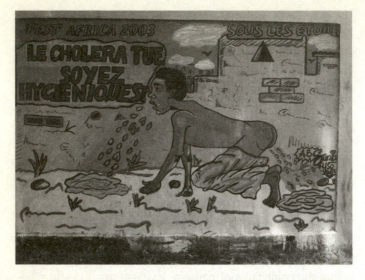

2. In early accounts, continuous vomiting was as important a symptom as uncontrollable diarrhea. (*Integrated Regional Information Networks, UN Office for the Coordination of Humanitarian Affairs*)

Some emphasized the vomiting. That put cholera in the class of a bilious colic, which in turn linked it to lead poisoning, another colic. Some, highlighting the end-stage cardiovascular effects, referred to a *cholera asphyxia*. Others, emphasizing the spasms, linked it to tetanus.

Pathological theories sometimes underlay this divergence. Seeing the key issue as the cause of the spasms and the expulsions from mouth and anus, the eminent Edinburgh systematist William Cullen put cholera in the neuroses.[4] (Classical writers had seen the spasms as the "choleric passion," noted James.) James, a mechanical philosopher, appealed directly to atoms. The acridity of bile itself might cause "racking, pungent, lancinating, corroding, and biting Pains" leading to convulsions.

He sought to explain why evacuation continued after the bile had presumably been expelled. James explained that spasming attracted humors. Juices flowed into the intestines and stomach and were kept from returning by the constriction of the veins. In similar manner James accounted for ulceration, inflammation leading to necrosis, and the sympathetic spread of the spasm to all parts of the body: together, the immediate causes of cholera.

Might we read James's humors as electrolytes, and see here a primitive account of the cholera toxin? To do so would miss the special flavor of these eighteenth-century attempts to access hidden pathological processes. That flavor, it has been often complained, was overly verbose—a rich vocabulary of atoms, fibres, nerves, or humors was allowed to substitute for observed fact. Yet there was more than speculation here. Well before the golden age of pathological anatomy in early nineteenth century Paris, cholera cadavers were finding their way to anatomists' tables remarkably often. In Europe, the anatomists Caspar Bartolin and Jean Riolan were pioneers. In India, dissection became possible owing to the fact that dying English soldiers were far from their families (by contrast, there were Hindu proscriptions against it). During the second pandemic (1830–7), cholera would be so strongly associated with dissection by citizens in Paris, New York, and some English towns that it would be seen as no disease, but a mass poisoning undertaken by the doctors to obtain bodies to dissect.

And yet, both before and after 1817, anatomy failed to illuminate. There were disparate findings as there had been disparate theories. Many would make the essence of the disease an ulceration of the small intestine. Yet so powerful and rapid were the effects of cholera that it was hard to distinguish primary from secondary features, or pathological effects on the living body from post-mortem deterioration. In the view of modern writers, cholera is a lesion-less disease: cholera toxin may drain the body but it leaves no visible holes.

So much for pathology; what of remote causes? Cholera, unlike dysentery, was rarely seen as contagious. It was an idiopathic event, or an accompaniment of another disease. It was, quite often, attributed to something one had eaten. That something might be a mineral poison. The symptoms of cholera were similar to those of an overdose of a strong mineral medicine, such as an antimonial compound. James cites a case in which arsenic was found in the gut of a cholera victim. His emphasis on acridity draws on the heritage of mineralogical chemistry: for early eighteenth-century medical chemists not only knew what such powerful reagents did, they thought they knew what they were—sharp atoms, for example. Since these poisons produce cholera-like symptoms, one may infer that whatever other entities cause cholera act in a similar manner. After 1817, medical writers would continue to stress the toxicological as opposed to pathological character of cholera; communities perceiving themselves as victimized by cholera would take the analogy in another direction and conclude that they were being poisoned.

The view of cholera as due to something you ate was one means of linking it to other digestive problems. In such classifications, cholera usually fell between ordinary diarrhea and dysentery. Even the "old" cholera differed from ordinary diarrhea in its rapidity and violence. Dysentery, on the other hand, was longer lasting and more serious, and likely to be epidemic. Usually it implied blood in the stool, but some referred to a non-bloody dysentery, which John Macpherson, one of the early cholera historians, would interpret as European cholera (*cholera nostras*) in epidemic form.

To say what foods were likeliest to cause a cholera was difficult. Fruit, particularly under-ripe acid fruit, was a particular worry. James lists "Melons, Pumpions, Cucumbers, Pine-apples, Peaches, Prunes, Grapes, Cherries," but also buttery cakes, and "Sweet-meats, Funguses, the Spawn of the Barbelfish, Must, New Wine, and Ale, and too fat Fleshes." But the concern was not only with the particular foods one ate but also with the whole context of eating: the mix of food and drink taken, the weather and the suitability of one's clothing to it (important with regard to the regulation of perspiration), the habits and more proximate activities of the partaker, and that person's own constitution. Flying into a rage after eating could trigger the disease even on a safer diet, like cabbage. One's rage after all might itself be a species of cholera; it too was an outpouring of bile. Bilious persons were to be particularly careful in their drinking habits; their overindulgence would upset the stability of the bile and "excite the most terrible Disorder in the Animal Economy." *Cholera infantum*, a severe infant diarrhea, could develop in this way too, when a mother's (or, presumably, a nurse's) passion was transferred to her milk "which assumes an Orgasm by the Passion, produces an Effervescence with the Bile in the delicate Stomach of the Infant, corrodes the Intestines, and generally gives occasion to a fatal Inflammation."[5]

This European classical cholera was not so different from concepts in other cultures. Classical Indian medicine, too, was broadly humoral; so too Chinese. Medical concepts in Islamic west Asia and north Africa were more conspicuously syncretic, but in all there were concerns with maintaining balance in the face of changing activity and climate. The constituents of balance were not identical. *Huo-luan*, the Chinese diagnostic category, would reflect concern with the hot–cold balance. In each culture, the terms that would include cholera were usually broader than the Hippocratic cholera or the new "Asiatic" cholera, but those terms also reflected different approaches to grouping symptoms, sometimes splitting what European concepts would lump. Cholera would be a site of contestation with regard to systems of therapy, but, even more importantly, to systems of prevention, and hygienic citizenship.

Therapy

"No theory is so gratuitous or absurd but cases may be found which appear to justify it," reflected a nineteenth-century cholera commentator.[6] Cholera therapy, equally for the old cholera and for the new, is often lampooned as desperate measures based on silly theories. It has been easy to ridicule cholera writers; they spent much ink ridiculing each other. But there were rationales and a long record of experience with the old cholera. Compared to most fevers, which had to be managed over their complex courses, cholera was simple: treat symptoms as they arise. There were three goals in cholera therapy, James explained: rid the body of the "peccant" matter; control the spasms; and restore strength. The first might take care of itself in the expulsive course of the disease. If that were not the case, very mild emetics (warm buttery water; broth) and/or purgative enemas, of whey, for example, might help. So too would absorbents (for example, easily digestible grains, as oats or rice). As antispasmodics, James, a classically trained physician, suggested a range of exotica starting with the "Liver of the Wolf dried," and "the Raspings of the Stag's Penis" or of the "human Cranium" and going on through various of the theriacs. (His successors and his predecessor Sydenham would almost invariably prescribe opium for this purpose, but it does not appear among James's suggestions.) Strengthening and toning were to be achieved by other herbals, but also by "Broths prepar'd with Veal, Fowls, the Roots of Succory, Parsley, Sparrow-grass, Chervil, bruis'd Crab-fish and Lemon-juice." Throughout the disease waters were to be given, sometimes cold, sometimes warm. James warned that "Sallies of passion" must be avoided as they might trigger a relapse.

James, like his successors, listed remedies in the order they might be tried—if one did not stop spasms, the next might. Only rarely was venesection indicated (and then to deal with inflammation), but James did suggest cupping, to reduce inflammation in the stomach. Many of his successors suggested a modest bleeding at the beginning of treatment. It was a means of lowering the constitution that might slow the spasms. From about 1830 to 1860, bleeding would become common in Indian practice. The eminent medical statistician F. Bisset Hawkins cited results of cholera practice from an East India company surgeon in 1818: only 2 of 88 patients who were bled died, but 8 of 12 who were not bled died.[7]

Most of James's remedies focus directly on symptoms. They dealt both with what hurt—coldness and cramping, heart-burn—and with what endangered, like the passing of watery stools, painless but worrisome. Within the holism of classical medicine, the experience of pain was less distinct from the diseased processes than it sometimes is in modern medicine. Warm baths, hot (even boiling) waters, and oils, or particular techniques of friction, might, by easing pain, also break the tension in other parts of the body. The antispasmodics were often anodynes as well; counter-irritants were, if not exactly ano-dynes, a means to move the spasms away.

We now recognize that cholera, like almost every other form of severe diarrhea, can be managed simply by replacing the lost fluids and salts, normally by oral rehydration. Most eighteenth-century physicians recognized that too. Their tactics differed. The comforting backup of intravenous intervention was not practicable, though it would be tried repeatedly in the nineteenth century, but most saw the value of water and decoctions or broths that are easily digestible or absorbent. The biochemistry was not yet of substances lost, but of sharp things needing to be dulled: softeners were whey, water, "lean broth, or small beer."[8] But the great problem in treating cholera was not in recognizing the need for fluids but in getting them to stay down. "Keep trying," we now say; use an IV if needed. Eighteenth-century doctors too gave the same advice, but did not have an IV as a backup. The preparations to be ingested might be varied, or administered by clyster, an instrument for injecting a large enema or purge.

And yet, without unambiguous warrant in the pathological theories that should guide treatments (for example, direct measures of fluid loss), they lacked confidence to push them hard in the face of failure. The grand dilemma of early medicine was the proper place of theory. A correct theory could suggest therapies and provide the confidence to push past initial failures; wrong theory led to the killing of patient after patient while supposedly getting the details right. The dilemma is at the heart of retrospective critiques of cholera therapy. They should have stuck with fluid replacement despite failure, we say; thrown out bleeding, despite apparent successes.

James's digest of learned medicine over the ages was tied to no single theory. After 1817, the virulence of the "new" cholera, together with the failure of old therapies, would put a premium on finally finding the essential pathological process, from which effective therapeutics could be derived. Often the theorists strayed far from symptom-based treatments to what would be seen as the therapeutic absurdities characteristic of cholera, all the work of an *idée fixe*. If a little did something, a lot would do more; hence a modest tactical anti-inflammatory bleeding could evolve into a dogma of "copious bleeding" based on the assumption of cholera as a form of blood poisoning. We may say that they thought too much, but blind empiricism is no satisfactory alternative either.

Prognoses varied. James was among the most pessimistic. With the exception of plague and pestilential fevers, "no Disease is more acute, or kills the Patient sooner, than a Cholera." Another admitted that "the [cholera] patient sinks sometimes in twenty-four hours." Cholera's greater dangerousness was part of the way it was distinguished from normal diarrhea. Most agreed that, if caught early, cholera could be cured quickly. Much depended on the victim's constitution and previous state of health. But even in the strong, it was sometimes fatal within a few hours. For James Lind, famous for his insights into scurvy, it made all the difference whether the disease arose in a healthy person or in a weakened one:

> The distinction necessary to be made between fluxes in all climates is,—That those which attack persons in perfect health may be considered in light of what physicians term original diseases; but those fluxes which attack persons very much weakened by a fever, and reduced to a very low condition of body, are properly symptomatic, as they proceed chiefly from the patient's debility and weakness…[9]

Well into the nineteenth century it would be argued that the variability of patients accounted for the differential effectiveness of therapies, and the need for expert care in cholera.

Cholera also varied by place and by time. By James's writing in the mid-eighteenth century, the old cholera was already recognized as endemic in India, Mauretania, Arabia, and America. Usually, geography was reduced to climate. The approach was long-standing. It was expected that there would be physiological and psychological responses to change of season that might require a dose of well thought out physick. In north-western Europe, respiratory diseases and pleurisies came in late winter and spring (we still speak of "flu" season), while diarrheas were autumnal. Cholera was expected from August through October. Thus John Huxham's summary for August 1735: "Many afflicted with Cholera and Diarrhoea. A great Number of Persons are greatly dispirited and listless from the untoward, wet, heavy Season. Many dogs run mad."

Choleras that took place in those months required little further explanation; those that did not could be attributed to autumn-imitating factors. By the end of the eighteenth century, many located these factors in barometric variations. Perhaps the humors were kept in hydrostatic balance by air pressure. The rapid changes of autumn might stir them up. Climate also proved a means to understand the differences between the cholera of Europe and that of India and the tropics. The tropics were just like Europe in the dog days of summer, only more so. Benjamin Rush noted that *cholera infantum* began in July in hot and humid Philadelphia. In even hotter Charleston, it began in April. Rush believed that its frequency and severity were a function of heat. It was the same disease as adult cholera; children got it first because they were more sensitive to temperature.[10]

And, finally, the old cholera came in epidemics. Thomas Willis's description of the non-bloody London dysentery of 1670 would often be cited.

The disease invading suddenly and frequently without any manifest occasion, did reduce those labouring with it by great vomiting, frequent and watery stools (excretory convulsions, with tormenting perturbation of the whole body) quickly to a very great debility, to horrid failure of the spirits, and a loss of all strength. I knew some, the day before well enough, and very strong, in twelve hours' space so miserably cast down…that with a weak and small pulse, cold sweat, short and quick breath, they seemed just ready to die.

The epidemic, said to kill up to 500 per week, lasted a month, typical of cholera's residence times in nineteenth-century cities. But it did not spread, and Willis saw no evidence of contagion. When, in the early 1870s, cholera became irreversibly Asian, this rich record of cholera-like epidemics in European towns—Nîmes in 1544, Mantua in 1564, Ghent in 1665, a number of English towns in 1669–76, and many outbreaks in the eighteenth century—would be reviewed but dismissed.[11] True cholera came from Asia; this must be some other disease.

One may wonder what any of this generic gastroenteritis has to do with the real cholera. Certainly it is important to cholera's history; it may be important to its pathology as well. Response to the new disease was framed in terms of the old. Even the concept of two distinct diseases misleads. Within the framework of constitutional medicine, diseases were defined in terms of positions along several continua rather than as products of unique infectious agents (the concept was analog, not digital). The new disease was only newish; it was sufficiently old to share the old name. No matter how often European physicians might hear in the early 1830s that the coming visitation was of a different cholera, they could not escape its old name, or jettison experience.

In fact, its newness would be contested well past mid century. During the century, that post-1817 disease would get newer and newer to Europe, at the same time as it was getting older to Asia. The identification of a microbe agent that was causing cholera in Egypt, India, and France in 1883–4 privileged change over continuity. It would be read as confirming the verdict of a new disease in 1817, though it could do so only indirectly.

That new disease, or, retrospectively, the first pandemic, began in August 1817, in Jessore in the Ganges delta, then forest covered and tiger riden, after unusually heavy rains. Having killed 10,000 persons there (it is claimed), cholera moved on to Kolkata in September. But it was a November outbreak among the military near Allahabad, 1,000 kilometers upstream on the Ganges, that would be seized upon by many later chroniclers. This was in an army of 10,000, but with 80,000 camp followers. Within a few days, 5,000 had died. "Before or since there is not any instance upon record," boasted the Indian army surgeon turned cholera writer James Kennedy, "in which the comparative mortality has been so extensive."[12]

Later writers would chart the pandemic as having moved first slowly and then more quickly, north-west into the Punjab and south-east into the Indonesian archipelago by 1820. By 1821 it had reached Oman at the southern tip of Arabia. Over the next two years it moved northward along the west shore of the Persian Gulf as well as overland through Teheran to the south shore of the Caspian Sea. By 1822 it had also reached Japan, the coastal trading ports of China (Canton), and far inland in eastern Siberia. Then it stalled, in 1823 or 1824. It had reached Russian territory at Astrakhan, but not European Russia. Some would collapse this first pandemic into the second; cholera had perhaps only paused in its advance on Europe.

How the "new" cholera became old

Was this a new disease in India or an old one? There was no reason why India, like every other place, should not have its cholera, but this disease would come to be seen as a unique Bengali invader. That Asianizing took place in two phases. Before 1840 the new cholera was accidentally Indian, a version of the universal *cholera morbus*, which just happened to strike India first on its way around the world. By the 1870s, that new disease was essentially and eternally Indian. Despite having been doubted by most who have carefully studied the issue, that view prevails today.

When East India Company surgeons began in the eighteenth century to practice their craft among the troops and traders in South Asia, they encountered new diseases, some of which affected delicate Europeans differently from locals—though that was hard to gauge, since their practice among these others was occasional and unrepresentative. Within the dominant Hippocratic framework, it was assumed that place modified bodily processes; it made sense to think that local practitioners knew best how to respond. Throughout the eighteenth and well into the first half of the nineteenth century European practitioners, French as well as English, would seek local knowledge of cures. They found multiple communities of healers, Muslim and Hindu, familiar with a disease that was most commonly known in Arabic as *haiza*, or as *mordesheen* in Mahrattan. (The latter term evolved into *mort du chien*, though it had nothing to do with dying dogs, and even into *Merde chi*—it certainly did have to do with *merde*.) In many cases, their techniques, and the principles that apparently underlay them, were similar to European therapies for *cholera morbus*. Calomel, the "Sampson of medicine," that would become the mainstay of mid-nineteenth-century cholera cures ("the only remedy that can cope with that enemy of life") was already well established in India.[13] And hardly surprisingly. The familiar humoral framework, the uses of mercurials and other heavy metals, reflected millennia of medical syncretism, of both theory and technique, from south-eastern Europe across most of Asia, and including China, a topic that would fascinate the cadre of late-nineteenth-century German philologists.

Strategies to redress the balance of humors, stop spasms, and support recovery were also similar. Tastes and smells were more central in Indian than in European medicine, evident in the use of spices and camphor. Essential oils were also much used, and seemed strikingly effective as specifics. They would be studied in twentieth-century clinical reviews but dismissed: their effectiveness seemed impossible to square with a bacteriological paradigm. External treatments to restore heat and ease spasms were also prominent. Mainly these were warm baths and friction, but they also included cauterizing the callused heel and ligating the limbs. That therapeutic theme would continue to be expressed in the issuing of flannel cholera belts to British Indian army. To promote recovery, Indian healers gave acidic drinks and rice gruel (now an important adjunct to oral rehydration).

Those relating south Asian cholera therapies did sometimes revel in the exotic. R. H. Scoutetten passed on a story from the earlier nineteenth-century French surgeon Gravier of the cure of a cholera sufferer in Pondicherry. A paste of lemon juice, alum, and iron oxide was rubbed over the man's eyes.

> The pain it produced vexed and enraged the sick man, and he attempted to strike those around him; the vomitings became more frequent, his attendants fled to avoid his blows; he pursued them; passing by a reservoir of water, which served

for the purposes of the garden, he plunged into it and drank with avidity for several moments. They surrounded him, but he remained tranquil in the water. The enormous quantity of liquid he drank, was followed by fainting. He was then removed from the reservoir and put to bed; he slept for eleven hours. When he awoke, the vomitings and dejections had ceased, but he was blind. This fact is known by all the inhabitants of Pondicherry.

Yet Scoutetten was not broadcasting the oddities of the east, but urging the need for rehydration; he noted that Gravier, his source, had "learned from an Indian doctor, named Rassendren, a very sensible man, that individuals who drank fresh water, recovered."[14] Respect of indigenous healing was such that, in setting up a training program for Indian practitioners in the 1820s, the Bengal administrators developed a curriculum based on both ancient Sanskrit texts and European authors and techniques.

All this belonged to what is sometimes seen as a golden age of toleration. So long as the East India Company's mission was extraction not rule, there was occasion for comprehension, appreciation, and respect, and sometimes for indulgence, encouragement, and cooptation of Indian religious, philosophical, as well as medical and administrative structures. By the second third of the century that toleration was falling before the evangelizing liberalism of Macaulay and the Mills. By the final third, imperial rule had become a matter of destiny not convenience. Indigenous medicine along with Indian culture more generally were superstitions to be tolerated where necessary to maintain order, but eradicated everywhere else.

Medicine, increasingly under the auspices of a universalizing biomedical science, might seem to belong unproblematically to the domain of technical matters that could be reformed. Not so. Medicine (and health) were bound up with Indian religions far more intimately than was the case in Europe. Brandishing the dichotomy of God *or* nature, the British could not fathom that spiritual and material might inhere in a single medical system. Hence a discourse of difference arose where universality might have been expected. In 1857, contempt for Hindu and Muslim practice had led to revolution. Thereafter, Empress Victoria would guarantee freedom of belief and practice, but colonial administrators learnt the lesson too well: in the case of sanitation at Hindu festivals, non-interference with religion led to neglect of public hygiene and to repeated outbreaks of cholera. Indigenous medicine might still be indulged; it need not be respected. In the 1860s, John Murray, a Bengal medical officer, noted the widespread use by English practitioners of a cholera pill of opium, black pepper, assefetida, and local herbs and spices. It was based on Indian practice. While English doctors would have concocted something similar, its acceptability to the native population was a significant part of its warrant.

The consolidation of cholera as Asian came as part of the post-1857 exoticizing of India. Increasingly, what had happened in 1817 would be looked upon not as novel event, but as eternal return. The conclusion that cholera was as ancient as Asia followed, but had relatively little to do with, the study of classical Indian medical texts. Physician-philologists were few enough; and earlier scholars of ancient Hindu medicine had not been particularly interested in cholera. Still, in the decade after 1817 some had broached the question of how new was this newish cholera. "In the medical works of the Hindoos," wrote the Madras surgeon Whitelaw Ainslie in 1825, "there are various disorders distinguished by violent vomiting, purging, sinking of the powers of life, &c., &c.... It is difficult ... to ascertain which may be considered as the real Cholera Morbus."[15] Summarizing the scholarship in 1831, Francis Bissett Hawkins noted that the key terms in the ancient texts were *Sitanga* and *Vidhuma Vishúchi*. Yet an account of the latter failed to mention vomiting and purging. It focused on the subjective: pains and griping, effects on vision and the intellect, faintness, thirst, and coldness. That focus might be due to perverse Asian epistemic standards, but Hawkins could not be sure. The deadly *Sitanga* seemed less ambiguous in its reference to vomiting and looseness but was a longer-lasting disease than cholera. As in European traditions, eating bad fruit was a cause. Neither description indicated a prehistory of pandemics. Writing a generation later, Scoutetten complained that earlier translators had extracted cholera-like symptoms from composite disease entities. In original context, these looked even less like cholera.

Making cholera Asiatic: a double Mac

The two authors chiefly responsible for the Asianizing of cholera were physician-historians who were not linguists. Both John Macpherson (1817–90) and N. Charles Macnamara (1832–1918) had achieved high rank in the Indian Medical Service and became cholera authors on retirement to England. Macpherson's *The Annals of Cholera from the Earliest Times to 1817* (1872) relied on R. H. Scoutetten's 1869 *Histoire chronologique topographique et étymologique du Choléra*, the first edition of August Hirsch's *Handbuch der historisch-geographischen Pathologie* (1859–64), and in key places on Macnamara's *Treatise on Asiatic Cholera* (1870). Then, in his *History of Asiatic Cholera* (1876), Macnamara relied on Macpherson. Hirsch drew heavily from both in his second edition (1881–3), which, in turn, would be the key source for Pollitzer in the 1950s, and thus the source for most modern claims that epidemic cholera has always been in Asia.

Their story is a mix of farce and prejudice. Briefly, Macnamara misread or misrepresented Macpherson, who was swayed by Macnamara's earlier gullibility. They held wholly incompatible concepts of what cholera was, but they seemed to be able to agree that it was eternally Asian, notwithstanding that both admitted that there was no *evidence* of epidemic cholera in ancient India.

Macpherson concentrated on the pre-1817 period, but did not independently review the ancient Indian texts. There were terms in Asian languages for cholera-like symptoms, but these did not clearly distinguish a definite disease entity, much less an epidemic one. "On the whole...the ancient writers on Indian medicine do not give nearly so clear and distinct an account of cholera as the Greek and Roman ones, and they afford no indication of any particularly virulent or epidemic form of the disease."[16] Macnamara followed: "The more carefully we study the writing of these early authorities...the clearer it appears that they had never met with cholera in its epidemic, or Asiatic form."[17]

Macpherson assumed that there was cholera in ancient India only because he assumed that there was cholera everywhere: it was, "in one shape or another...in all ages a world-wide malady." It came with "a variety of symptoms...[and] must have been...very familiarly known, for in Europe almost every country had a popular name for it, and in India there was not a district or a language, that had not its local name."[18]

Thus, if some sort of "cholera" had been always and everywhere, surely there had always been Asiatic cholera in Asia.

Had we any doubts, the Portuguese resolved them. They met cholera as soon as they reached India; surely it had been there before. If the accounts of European explorers were lacking in desired clinical precision, that was hardly surprising. Most were not medically trained; the exception was the seventeenth-century Dutch physician James Bontius, who described a disease that sounded like sporadic cholera. It killed so rapidly that poisoning was suspected. This Macpherson accepted as "the true malignant cholera," though it was not pandemic. Were there then two choleras? Macpherson is ambiguous. After 1500 we could "conveniently treat of cholera in the East, and cholera in Europe, separately, always recollecting that in all parts of the world it was *a disease of varying intensity*."[19]

Macpherson could be ambiguous because he was appealing to a clinical concept of disease. By 1884 he had reluctantly admitted that there might be a cholera germ ("if it is preferred to use that expression"), but the phenomena of cholera were so various that it explained nothing. Macpherson's two choleras were not the ones that later writers would distinguish: the real thing, caused by *Vibrio cholerae* O1, and the host of pretenders, anonymous gastroenteritises. The Asian cholera he could recognize after 1500 was distinct not in essence, but in virulence and epidemicity.

Why was Indian cholera so much more terrible? Maybe the patient and the patient's environment were responsible— Indian cholera was deadlier because its victims were weaker. By 1830 it was clear to most that the new cholera was linked to poverty. It might be seen as a proxy of poverty, an ordinary disease that got out of hand in dense and debilitated populations. Scoutetten wrote of "le genre de vie des Indiens," a matter of misery, improvidence, and the depressive action of heat, humidity, and temperature change. Later, colonial public-health officials would note the common coincidence of cholera with famine in India, but it remained coincidence.

There was only one clinical sign that *might* distinguish Asian from other cholera: bile. The European disease was classically conceived as an evacuation of yellow, green, or black bile, while the Indian disease would be known for a clear evacuation, the famed "rice-water" excretions (thus, some sticklers would deny "cholera" as the right name for the new disease).[20] Ultimately, the difference would be largely explained in terms of stage— once the gut had been cleansed, only the watery fluid was left. And there were plenty of records of watery discharges in the earlier European cholera: for example, "an aqueous and thin Liquour, which sometimes resembles the Washings of Flesh" (James); stools "nearly as limpid as water" (Rush). Through a point-by-point comparison of the supposed differences between *cholera morbus* and "malignant cholera," Macpherson himself would arrive at the modern view: severe non-cholera gastroenteritis is clinically indistinguishable from cholera.[21] (Ironically, as humoral theory waned, cholera pathology would be redefined in terms of bile retention: on dissection, the gall bladders of cholera victims were distended. Bile even became a cure. A traditional remedy in India, it would later be shown to kill microbes in cholera stools.)[22]

For Macnamara, disease essences were permanent, but not universal. He held an etiological concept of disease. He reinterpreted Macpherson's infinite variation as dichotomous difference. The deadly beast from the east, a uniquely Indian, inherently deadly, pandemic disease, was wholly distinct. All else was the friendly and familiar *cholera nostras*. Macnamara was a proponent of John Snow's theory of cholera as a specific water-borne disease and a defender of Robert Koch's bacteriology. He invoked a logic of reciprocal justification. A single species of germ produces a distinct disease; we read accounts of epidemics to single out instances of that distinct disease, which then warrant the assumption of a single germ. This, along with a large dose of racialized epistemology, led to the conclusion that the "new" disease, severe epidemic cholera, had *always* been in India.

The overlooking of epidemic cholera was no accident. Ancient Indian culture *must* fail to recognize such epidemics: its medicine was one of traditionalism and sacred texts not empiricism or induction; its focus on the elite would deflect attention from the diarrhea of the masses. Finally, India's (supposed) social, cultural, and economic insularity in ancient times would have impeded both the spread of the disease and the opportunity to recognize it by learning from other cultures. It took cosmopolitan inductive Europeans to recognize cholera, to problematize it, and to solve the problem. Global cholera was simply an unfortunate by-product of bringing India into the world. Macnamara wrote that his book would be "an account of a controllable disease which has within the last fifty years burst forth from British India; and destroyed on each occasion millions of human beings, many of them in the prime of life; and all cut off by this malady have endured frightful agony during the few hours they have lingered in its grasp."[23]

Should anyone doubt the antiquity of cholera, Macnamara had a clincher. There was a Hindu cholera deity, the goddess Oola Beebee (or Ola Bibi), worshipped in lower Bengal, precisely the home of the cholera. Goddess-creation was demand-driven: "It seems…certain that the malady must have raged at times with violence, or it would not have been found necessary to propitiate the Deity specially on account of it." Macpherson too was convinced. That creation, moreover, was assumed without question to be the work of a distant past.[24] Both knew that the shrine to Oola Beebee was new in 1818, but assumed it must be a revival of the cult of an ancient goddess. Traditional societies were, after all, "traditional." Oola Beebee is not in standard versions of the Hindu pantheon. That religion might be adaptive did not occur to these orientalists. In the twentieth century, the eminent Kolkata pathologist S. N. De looked into the matter. He concluded that Oola Beebee was not revived but created by a shrine entrepreneur. Macnamara and Macpherson had also conflated shrines to Sheetolla or Sitala, a smallpox goddess, with the cholera goddess.

For Macnamara and Macpherson, cholera was an Indian disease, but a European concept, a product (and vindication) of observation. But what happened when Europeans failed to notice it? That question arose after 1817, particularly with regard to disease outbreaks in the early 1780s, but also as early as 1761–2, when a cholera-like disease is said to have killed 30,000 natives and 800 Europeans in Bengal. The 1781–2 epidemic was a rapidly fatal disease of vomiting, purging, and spasms that first broke out in an East India Company force of 5,000. The mortality is not recorded, but 1,143 were hospitalized, and Jameson, the most commonly cited source, estimated 700 deaths. It was attributed initially to poisoning, then to bad water. It spread to Kolkata, where the eminent Warren Hastings reported at least 879 deaths in ten days, then north-east to Sylhet and south, reaching Madras in late 1782 and affecting French south India as well. In 1783 it killed an estimated 20,000 pilgrims to Hardiwar, upstream on the Ganges. Hastings himself likened it to the *cholera morbus* of Europe. Yet, though recurring through the 1790s, it would become unworthy of remark, just another of the many diseases of hot climates and of the strange peoples who lived in them. Hastings's observation was forgotten. What began in 1817 *seemed* new. Had movement to the south-east been weighted equally with movement to the north-west, we might well recognize an Asian pandemic from 1761 to 1804, which extended north and east to Burma and China, south to Sri Lanka, and west to Mauritius.

Feeling a need to explain why the Company's medical officers had missed all this, Macnamara concluded that they were ruled by bad theory and that control of India was incomplete. Even in areas of company control, record-keeping was not what it might have been, and as for areas outside it, no one could hope to know what was going on there.

But there was another anomaly. In the view that would ultimately prevail, cholera came from Bengal. But the reports of Indian choleras before the mid eighteenth century were from almost everywhere *but* Bengal. There were outbreaks well south along the Coromandel coast, but most were from the west, from Mumbai, south to Goa, sites of European trading missions. Again, the anomaly was blamed on records; cholera was reported when Europeans were there to report it. Yet cholera would be constructed as Bengali, and in the process Bengali people, chiefly men, were effectively "niggered": made the blackest of the blacks, and effeminate to boot.[25] Pollitzer's handling of the issue in 1955 suggests how much creative reinterpretation had gone on: "the known early history of cholera in India furnishes hardly any clue for the cardinal epidemiological importance of Bengal, which, according to the present state of our knowledge, has to be considered as the cradle, if not the original home, of the infection...[Yet] observations made in that area from 1817 onwards filled this gap...in so dramatic a manner that some of the observers were led to believe that the disease had then arisen in Bengal *de novo*."[26]

Thus cholera is exoticized. Everything fits. In the mysterious east, epidemics kill masses, yet for millennia never rise to consciousness. But of course. Since Asians are fatalistic and undervalue individual lives, they *would* not notice; that they *do* not becomes proof that there was cholera *to be* noticed. Sadly, however, the rest of the world must suffer from their failure to face their own problems (and the British government's failure to make them do so).

Blameworthy pandemics?

Such was the view of cholera epidemiology that August Hirsch accepted in the early 1880s. Cholera came from India (he would call it "*cholera Indica*"). Any association with the sporadic *cholera nostras* represented "a mistake in diagnosis...the confounding of two forms of the disease, which certainly approach one another closely in the matter of symptoms, but, as regards their origin and clinical history, have nothing in common." The spreading cholera killed about half it struck; the "so-called *cholera nostras*" did not spread and rarely killed. Ancient Hindu writings or travelers' accounts were not to be trusted fully, but a record of epidemic cholera from the late 1760s was clear. Within India cholera was regional, the Bengal anomaly due to poor records.[27]

Most importantly, the conviction that cholera came always from India allowed Hirsch to conceive the cholera "pandemic." A sequential pattern of outbreaks might be read as the communication of cholera; that recognition of (apparent) communication of some cholera from Bengal led to the conviction that all cholera must come from Bengal. More than the cholera of the 1780s, or that of 1817–24, it would be the second pandemic, beginning in 1829, that would be paradigmatic. Cholera covered much of Europe and crossed the Atlantic. Again Bengal is seen as the source; again movement was both eastward (a reinfection of Singapore, and then a move northward to Japan and Peking), and to the west, into Punjab by 1827, and north, reaching Moscow in 1830. After the Russian army had carried it to Poland, cholera moved west in 1831, and south-east to Constantinople. Caught by Muslim pilgrims, it moved south into Africa. Having reached the north of England via the Baltic trade by the end of 1831, it crossed to Canada and thence to the United States by the summer of 1832. Filtering into western Europe by several routes, it was in Paris by March 1832 and Spain by 1833. It may have reached South America.

Or so the retrospections went. In several cases routes of transmission were speculative. Rumors of outbreaks were rife, so too denials; and outbreaks of various epidemics, bowel-related or not, might be read as cholera. In subsequent epidemics, questions about routes of transmission would be supplemented by questions of whether outbreaks represented new introductions—again a journey of some entity outward from Bengal—or the recrudescence, due to unknown causes, of existing foci of infection. That there were often discrepant views as to just how and when cholera had reached a particular place (and even whether it had gotten there at all) did not dent the generalization: all cholera came from Bengal.

Through Hirsch, the voices (though not the reservations) of Macpherson and McNamara have prevailed. Pollitzer would accept the existence of cholera in India "since immemorial times" and agree with Macnamara that "irrefutable proof" came from the Portuguese and Dutch accounts. He acknowledged the difficulty of distinguishing pandemics from one another, and of distinguishing the first from the preceding epidemiological regime. Most have followed Pollitzer, in the process ignoring pre-1830s European choleras while acquiescing in loose translations across multiple languages.

A counter-narrative exists but does not go as far as it might. In it, "Asiatic" cholera remains eternally Asian, but colonizers are responsible for moving it after 1817: "Global movements carried a local gastroenteritis attack to Europe and America and reenacted the double fears of the plague and the attack of the Mongol hordes," notes Vijay Prashad.[28] This "Asiatic Cholera" is a new entity, only because it is a colonial entity. Nineteenth-century writers had recognized that the eighteenth-century outbreaks were associated with troop movements; indeed, they write often of the "march" of cholera. In later pandemics, the very trade routes Macnamara celebrated were seen as routes of transmission. To those writers, recognition had not implied apology: troop movements and trade were necessary, unlike, as we shall see later, pilgrimage.

To those writers, it was not the moving, but the source of what was moved, that was held responsible for cholera; that relegation now seems arbitrary and unfair. French writers had been more critical. Why no epidemics before 1817, asked Scoutetten—because the English were not moving about the country. (French colonizers surely would not have spread cholera, had they prevailed.) Indian criticisms that the new cholera was a product of colonization simply did not register: they were presented in a religious idiom. By camping in sacred groves, ignoring caste prohibitions, the troops had undermined cosmic and hygienic order.

What really happened?

Usually we consider two alternatives: (1) that real cholera was indigenous to Asia (Bengal), and colonialism and commerce brought it to the rest of the world; or (2) that a new disease, or a newly virulent strain of cholera, arose in Bengal in the mid-eighteenth century. The two are not mutually exclusive, since the latter allows that an older cholera might have evolved.

Most have dismissed the European cholera. Pollitzer, and more vehemently Norman Howard-Jones, were sure that it was not the same thing. Whether or not it is true, the reigning model is based on asymmetric interpretive practices of nineteenth-century writers. European outbreaks are excluded on lack of epidemicity; Asian sources are included without evidence of it. Epidemics that early modern Europeans called cholera, which had the symptoms of cholera, were (are) varieties of gastroenteritis. Ambiguous gut diseases from south Asia are presumed to be the work of *Vibrio cholerae*. Macnamara is significantly responsible.

Always there were dissenters. Howard-Jones thought they had been misled by taking the word "cholera" for the thing. That is implausible. Many—De, Creighton, Winslow—were cholera experts or eminent epidemiologists. Recent recognition of multiple loci of autocthonous *Vibrio cholerae* (to be discussed in the Chapter 6) gives their views renewed plausibility.

Yet, by the usual logic of epidemiology, it is possible to go further. If there is no clear evidence of cholera in Asia before colonization, and if we know there were "cholera" epidemics in Europe in the sixteenth century, we might infer that the colonizers brought it. If commerce explained cholera in the nineteenth century, why not earlier? Once the Portuguese had come, the Indian Ocean became a busy place for European shipping. Before reaching India, ships would often have stopped at Zanzibar or at Aden or Muscat on the Arabian coast; there was ample possibility for picking up a disease in one place and putting it down in another. Macpherson does muse: "If we have no notice of cholera before the arrival of the Europeans, and then only of its prevalence in the parts visited by them..." Yet he goes on to the unsupported conclusion that "it is surely probable, not only that the disease was to be found in India before their arrival, but also that it was not limited merely to the districts with which they communicated." Again the issue is competent observation. "In the sixteenth century we have thus found cholera to have been present in Western India only, but, be it remarked, in the only places where Europeans had any opportunity of observing the diseases of the country."[29]

I do not say this happened. Yet it is well to keep in mind how much meager evidence was stretched and plausible inferences made into certainties. Epidemiological reconstruction in infectious diseases is not, and cannot be, a form of independent induction; if it were, it would be limited by the fallacious logic of post hoc, propter hoc. Invariably (and appropriately) it is informed by theory—pathology, microbiology, and the clinical sciences. The long-standing view of cholera as exclusively endemic to Bengal supported one chain of inference; the more recent view of *Vibrio cholerae* as a widely distributed marine organism of varying virulence supports another.

The theories have implications. The former reinforced a view in which Europeans suffered only from a friendly and manageable *cholera nostras*, while fatalistic and superstitious Asians, caring little for human lives, wallowed in their own filth and distributed it as deadly cholera, throughout the globe. The latter depicts cholera once again as universal, if, in some ways, as disturbingly accidental: no one is to blame for an obscure member of a plankton ecosystem. Both versions remind us that cholera must *mean*, not merely at a broader level at which symbolic associations are formed in particular cultures, but at a narrower one at which inductions are made guides for action.

II

⁓

CHOLERA FINDS ITSELF

I n the thirty-three quatrains of execrable verse of *The Chaunt of the Cholera* (1831) the Irish poet-playwright-novelist John Banim (1792–1842) treats the coming cholera as a vindicator of liberalism. Cholera is a matter as much of culture as of culture plates. It was no mere disease, but a signifier. Poetry is a key medium of meaning-making (especially in the Romantic age); cholera generated scads of the stuff. Banim's, in which personified cholera "smites," is one of the better known.

It is the European cholera of 1831–2 that created the meaning cholera still has: brash and bad, coming to get *you*, especially a readily victimizable "you." In looking back at the *cholera nostras* of earlier centuries, one is struck by *how little* the disease meant. It was dangerous, sometimes deadly, occasionally epidemic, yet warranted only a gloss in medical texts—dress warmly, avoid fruit in the autumn.

In many parts of the world—but not all—this new cholera raised issues of justness and accountability. Cholera and colds are both preventable communicable diseases. We *catch* a cold; cholera *strikes*—the dirty, ignorant, or profligate—or invades the poorly guarded town or nation. Rosenberg puts it well: "to die of cholera was to die in suspicious circumstances."[1] It is there

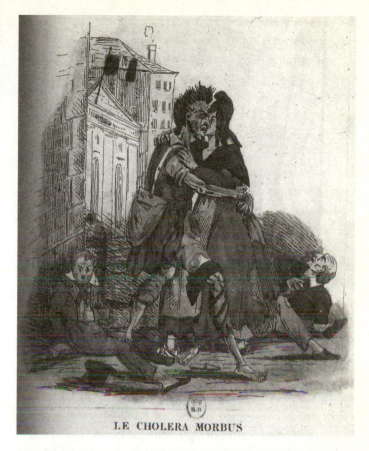

LE CHOLERA MORBUS

3. In this anti-liberal cartoon, cholera thanks the July revolutions (and such nationalisms in general) for helping it spread. Without the French and Polish revolutions it would still be stuck in Russia. (*Visages du Cholera*)

for a reason; "don't take it personally" won't work when one is hearing precisely the opposite on every frequency. Ironically, attempts to make cholera just another disease, a result of flawed environment or minute pathogen, almost always backfired. What was supposed to be a universal message about amoral nature turned out to be divisive and accusatory. Blame-laying and meaning-making were ways of coping.

The meanings were not new, even if the disease might be. Cholera could be recruited into anyone's ideology. It could be counted on to wither pride, punish the wicked, enlighten the ignorant, recall apostates to righteousness; one had only to identify the membership of each of these groups. For Banim, it meant revolution and retribution; for Robert Southey reaction and retribution. As a destroyer of order, it was enlisted to enforce order; its immorality or amorality was to augment morality, since cholera was an unmistakable call for cohesion. It preyed on the weak; bound them to the strong. Then and still now, simply to shout "cholera" had a remarkable effect quite independently of whether any severe diarrheal disease actually showed up.

We think cholera should *mean*; it must for action to be taken. In inferring that Asians had suffered from cholera for generations unending without noticing it, Macnamara had denied that assumption. His racism is plain. The view that Indian cholera was of "demographic" significance only is denied by David Arnold, who insists that the 1817 outbreak *was* seen by Indians too as a novel catastrophe requiring explanation. A "cholera as normal" interpretation can be self-fulfilling, worry Charles Briggs and Clara Mantini-Briggs in their anthropological study of the 1992 Orinoco cholera.[2]

Even when we allow for differential access to the means of expression and protest (themselves attributes of modernity), it appears that cholera was not equally problematic everywhere. Often importance is out of step with incidence. While individual mortality figures may be untrustworthy, the common view (probably right) is that cholera was deadlier in Asia than in Europe and in eastern Europe than in western. But it is in

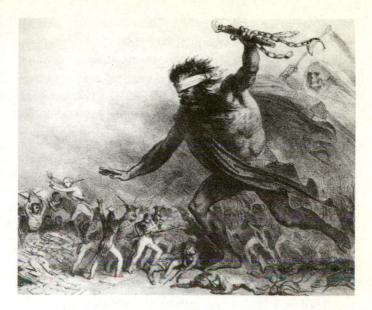

4. As in Banim's poem, cholera was often seen, especially in its first European experience, as a monster from the east. (*Visages du Cholera*)

western Europe that cholera appears to be most problematic. In Britain, hit lightly only by the second, third, and fourth pandemics, cholera is a central theme of nineteenth-century history.

Yet recurrent deadly disease can be normal. Plague and smallpox became so in early modern Europe. Where bowel diseases were regular, cholera might blend into the background of ordinary life or fail to rise above all the other epidemic and endemic ways of dying on offer. The Chinese response was negligible; the French or the Italian poor did not distinguish it, except in terms of the furor of the authorities; in England the cholera of 1848–9 killed more than twice as many as the earlier epidemic, but there was less sense of crisis. Not only the disease but what was problematic about it rose and fell and changed. We have no basis beyond a moral one to take the other extreme, to assume that *they* were just like *us*, individuals invested in self-determination and progress, and conclude therefore that cholera must have been a cosmic outrage. This is a tricky problem for a historian. Below I treat it as a problem of comparative theodicy, a matter of the politics of the permissibility of natural evils.

Who cares?

Much of the story of cholera in the nineteenth century is a story about who cares about it. Nowadays, everyone is expected to care, since cholera is a global problem. During the 1990s the mantra of microbial modernity was often heard: thanks to jet flights, *Vibrio cholerae* can get from the bowels of anyone to the mouth of anyone else in a few days. Thus, we are all brothers; in the cholera of each lies the potential cholera of all.

This is wishful thinking. Since the mid-nineteenth century, cholera has been an axis of difference, a means for distinguishing places and races as clean or dirty, and a vehicle for despising others. Cholera would be a disease of *them*, not *us*. Groups would be viewed in terms of presumed cholera status, as victims or as transmitters of the disease. Even as universalizing aspirations (for freedom from cholera) were being pursued, that pursuit was framed by writing off places, persons, and behaviors. The eventual eradication of a well-understood, preventable, and easily cured disease from some parts of the world only highlighted the fact that it persisted in other parts. Cholera remains "a leading means of sustaining Orientalism, the notion that peoples from North Africa, the Middle East, and Asia occupy a social realm that is forever alien, premodern, superstitious, and undemocratic," note Briggs and Martini-Briggs. Its power to divide is stronger than its power to unite.[3]

Our old *cholera nostras* had none of these qualities. How then did the new(ish) cholera gain them?

To a large degree, both the problematic character and the divisiveness arose with liberalism. In the world being imagined at the end of the eighteenth century, free and self-interested individuals would better themselves and, in doing so, better all. The partisans in the famous "conditions-versus-character" debate of 1840s England disagreed about whether failure to embody liberal habits and values was due to failed institutions or underperforming persons, but they agreed on a more important matter: the sort of "sanitary citizenship" that was required.[4] Both sides appealed to a concept of human capability that was the foundation of political, economic, and religious liberty, and national self-determination. Disease, on the other hand, eroded both the use and the exchange value of bodies, and blocked mechanisms of betterment. This set up a vicious cycle of poverty and hopelessness. Political freedom was predicated on biological freedom. Free persons might overcome natural challenges (cholera epidemics), but to do so they must be free of cholera epidemics.

So what of the actually or potentially choleraic? In effect, liberalism imposed an axis. Persons not white, Protestant, educated, wealthy, or male might ultimately bear liberal responsibilities and privileges, but at best their liberalization would come slowly and, perhaps, never completely. All who could not (even by non-liberal means) be made to meet the challenge of cholera belonged to a pre-modern residue best kept sequestered.

Liberalism did not issue fully grown from the thigh of Venus. Attacking in the fledgling years of liberalism, cholera helped to shape it. Buoyed up by Enlightenment ideals, liberals were unready for cholera. Hence the irritation of English radicals in 1832: here they were, finally getting Catholic emancipation and parliamentary reform only to have a novel epidemic worm its way onto the public agenda and call forth all manner of anti-quated dictatorial responses—cholera was surely a conservative job.

In other ways, too, the coincidence of the disease with contingent geographic, political, racial, economic, cultural, and institutional factors had far-reaching and unintended effects. Most important was that cholera was not home grown. Liberalizing Europe inherited it with all the east Indian entanglements of preceding centuries. The peevish racism little Mary exhibits in the opening pages of *The Secret Garden*—persons are either neglectful parents who try to deny her existence, an Indian nurse who is her closest attachment but entirely replaceable, or numberless Asians who "die like flies" or flee— had not been so pronounced when cholera was becoming restive a century earlier.

There is no need to add a racist element to the first cholera recognitions by Portuguese mariners: cholera, if that is what it was, was a strange disease in a strange land. Few of these explorer-marauder-traders were doctors. Often their accounts are big fish stories: they, or the hacks who rewrite their tales, are struck by (or seek out) the strange and remarkable. But they began a process. In the hands of Macpherson (and Macnamara), their stories would be one pillar of the edifice of an eternal, eastern cholera.

Race entered as a concomitant of the military contexts in which Europeans initially confronted cholera in India: cholera statistics came from East India Company regimental surgeons who customarily distinguished "Europeans" from "natives." These, along with officers and other ranks, were the categories in which human beings existed for James Annesley, a Madras regimental and hospital surgeon, who used them to assemble 31 tables covering over 100 pages, in a seminal work of 1825.[5] His findings were inconclusive as to whether race was a factor. Only rarely do the early writers seize on instances of the immunity of Europeans or of officers in a finger-waving way. When Bisset Hawkins writes that "while thousands of the latter [natives] were perishing by the epidemic in a district near Bombay, only six European soldiers died of it," he is reporting, not crowing.[6] Mostly the concern was with places that might be relatively healthy for Europeans, not in racial differences per se. The numbers were needed to compare places, by race and over time.

Among the few who probed such results was Reginald Orton, one time regimental surgeon of HM 34th Regiment of Foot, author of an *Essay on Epidemic Cholera* (1831). Orton noted that, while cholera morbidity (percentage of soldiers stricken) was significantly higher for Europeans, case mortality (percentage of stricken who die) was lower. Putting these statistics together showed an overall cholera mortality slightly lower for natives (5.25 per cent) than for Europeans (6.75 per cent). Race did not seem to matter much, but class (and culture) might. Of disease in general, he found that "the higher ranks...have been found in India to suffer less than the lower." Officers were generally stronger and better fed and clothed than their men, did not use "the common privies," and drank spirits steadily but temperately, rather than alternating between binging and water-drinking. Indian soldiers avoided alcohol, but lived on a poor rice diet and slept on the ground. Orton does not isolate factors of sanitation or water; all this together explains differential mortality.[7]

Given the prominence of Hippocratic explanations of health and disease, and equally the shock of south Asian heat and humidity to many Europeans, it is surprising how little the new cholera was explained in terms of the categories of tropical disease. That framework had been set out in James Johnson's popular *The Influence of Tropical Climates* (1813). It was expected that the health of Europeans would differ from that of natives. If Europeans suffered more, climate was to blame; if less, civilization and constitution were ascendant (impoverished Asians were less than fully alive in some representations). If Europeans succumbed soon after arrival, this was from failure to acclimatize; if they began in health but deteriorated, that was from progressively debilitating heat, humidity, or a new diet. If Europeans were relatively resistant, it was because they were better fed and more lightly worked.

Even if the focus on European versus native, and, behind it, military versus civilian, reflected bureaucratic blinders more than overt racism, those categories would carry over into later ideological regimes that were overtly racist. Moreover, ways of seeing were equally ways of not seeing, and they came at the expense of other demographic enquiries that, had they been taken up, might have proved useful in the elucidation of cholera. Soldiers and officers happened to be male; there was little attention to sex or to age. Orton reported that children were relatively immune from cholera and that it was particularly deadly for the aged. In Kolkata it was claimed that men were struck four times more often than women; elsewhere the difference was less, and in some places non-existent. Cholera was said to be particularly common and deadly for pregnant women, the spasms of cholera being likened to contractions. But all this was rumor or speculation; there was little hard evidence or interest in getting any. The inaccessibility of a large civilian population made it impossible even to consider a key question of whether, as with smallpox, recovery from cholera brought immunity. Orton, one of the few to address the topic, could study it only in the military; the civil population of India was too anonymous, untraceable, and indistinguishable.

The "natives" category also rendered India socially and culturally monolithic. Hindu and Muslim, caste, regional identity: rarely do these matters concern cholera authors even into the twentieth century. An exception, worth considering because of its prescient assessment of cultural factors in cholera, is James Christie's 1876 *Cholera Epidemics in East Africa*. Christie focuses on Zanzibar, where he spent several years as physician to the Sultan. Overall, he was appalled by the sanitary condition of "Stinkibar"on the usual moralizing grounds. The beach at night was the site of sex and defecation. There was no sanitary authority or medical police.

Rather, Zanzibar was a congeries of ethnic enclaves each self-governed by "custom."[8] Ethnic distinctions were multiple. Hindee Muslims from south Asia differed from south Arabians; among the former were groups distinct by regional origin or trade. Though intermingled within the city, these suffered the cholera epidemic of 1869–70 very differently. Europeans on ships suffered heavily, while shore-dwelling Europeans escaped, as did Banyans—a Hindu caste and the capitalists of Zanzibar. The Europeans escaped because they filtered their water; the Banyans escaped because of their rigorous hygienic isolation: they ate a simple vegetarian diet, cooked their own food, ate from disposable material (leaves), drank water from their own wells (and carried their own water when traveling), washed their own meager cotton clothing and their bodies daily, spent a half-hour daily cleaning teeth and tongue, plucked all body hair, defecated twice daily, and were quick to medicate incipient illness. (And yet, from a European standard, their dwellings were dirty, with dust and cobwebs, and they preferred to sleep in the odor of cow dung.) Other groups impressed Christie too. The Kohjahs, a Muslim group, had an extraordinary commitment to one another in sickness. All the Muslim groups followed Koranic hygienic commands, but to different degrees and in different ways.

There were also profound differences in water sources. The American consul had had samples analyzed; the results showed how far culture dictated "taste." Most water had to be carried in, but groups favored different sources. To wealthy Arabs waters were as important as wines to a European. They could distinguish waters by taste and blamed illnesses on bad waters. Europeans insisted that their servants fetch water from a distant spring, but were often served adulterated water from brackish nearby wells and could not tell the difference. Some Africans and some south Asian Muslims favored a whitish water, "something like diluted skim milk," with a "strong faecal smell," which was liked for its sweetness. It came from pits in the sand. Ships refilled from two streams, which were regular sites of defecation.[9]

Compared to standard Victorian sanitary distancing—a withering othering—Christie's recognition of hygiene as an arena of cultural expression is refreshing. He sees Zanzibar as an ecosystem of interacting communities, each occupying an economic, social, and hygienic niche. It thus constituted a natural experiment, one that showed that culture mattered more than place, and that cultures of water were particularly important. Though he blamed reliance on unhygienic black servants, refugees from many parts of Africa, for Zanzibar's health problems, he was not concerned with race as such. Rather, for Christie, analysis of cultural difference was to be a basis of prevention.

Social analysis had not always been undertaken in the context of prevention. Earlier Indian cholera writers had noted differential experience of cholera within the constraints of colonial, and more particularly military, institutions. Prophylactic implications were modest. The regimental surgeon might advise on camp hygiene and diet but was in no position to upset a military hierarchy defined as much in different psychological states of commanders and commanded as in different conditions and conveniences by rank and race. Similarly, it was apparent that Indian cholera provided, as Bisset Hawkins put it, "fresh confirmation of a most important principle in state medicine—that *the tendency to a fatal termination of disease increases in proportion to the poverty and ignorance of the individual.*"[10]

But these are facts, not problems. Poverty is not anomalous, problematic, or blameworthy: those liberal expectations had yet to be applied to India. Hawkins and Orton are not unsympathetic. Both admit that the plight of the poor may be improved at least temporarily. But, without undue hostility to victims or criticism of rulers, they come close to seeing cholera as a means of Malthusian equilibration. In a mysogenic moment, Orton observed that, in Bengal, cholera, "attacking chiefly the lowest class" as usual, "was particularly prevalent among the abandoned class of women." He cited a Chinese view: "the pestilence knew its victims."[11] Later in the century "Malthus" would not be respectable in polite company; but there would be greater antipathy to those dying of cholera (and spreading it) owing to heightened expectations of sanitary citizenship.

There were two additional incidental means of social division that cholera brought with it. They had to do with numbers and with minds.

Numbers

Any writer recording the new scourge of cholera quickly discovered that the polities hit by cholera could be readily divided between those which counted victims and those which offered only raw numbers. When cholera swept across India in the years after 1817, colonial officials relied on rumors or rough estimates of death tolls. Extrapolations from military to civilian deaths produced estimates as high as forty million Indian deaths during cholera's first fourteen years (Arnold estimates 1–2 million).[12]

That some populations can readily by counted, while others can only be estimated, is not inherently sinister, yet the difference between single digits and round numbers—often in units of tens of thousands—does suggest whether individual lives can matter: persons count when they can be counted and are required to be accounted for. When these conditions do not obtain, they die anonymously en masse.

There are inexplicable mixes of precision and imprecision. Scoutetten reports 10,000 deaths at Jessore in the first two months, but in Dacca 3,757 of 6,354 cholera patients died. At Sylhet, "of 3,316 houses, containing 18,896 inhabitants, in five months 10,000 were attacked with the cholera; of these 1,197 or one in eleven, died." A general pattern is clear, however: the move from Asia to Europe is from estimation to (pretended) precision. Thus 40,000 died in Bangkok in 1819; 60,000 in Muscat in 1821. Yet the record for Moscow, by November 10, 1830, was: 5,507 cases, 2,908 deaths.[13] In parading these figures, authors rarely cite sources, consider means of counting, or address the plausibility of the results.

Precision did not guarantee accuracy. The Canadian cholera writer Robert Nelson reported that there were 3,853 deaths in Montreal in the 1832 cholera. He obtained the figure by adding an estimate of 2,000 to the 1,853 officially recorded deaths.[14] Yet in doing so he was recreating the strong distinction between the civilized world of counting and accountability, and those mysterious places where untold numbers might perish. Even the presences of censuses did not assure accuracy. On the contrary, the appearance of precision was the most powerful instrument of deception, as the Italian government recognized in successfully denying the existence of epidemic cholera in 1911. Accountability might be predicated on countability, but the latter did not guarantee the former. Suspicions of statistical honesty could easily reinforce paranoia about mass poisonings by the state or about the grim and hidden things being done to untold numbers in cholera hospitals.

Still, the uncountable were in a worse situation. The well-known outbreak in the army near Allhallabad in 1817 was confusing, because it was not clear whether the figures were based on the army's recognized personnel or also included its enormous tail of camp followers and servants, usually estimated at eight times "strength." Thus, while the common figures are about 10,000 troops and 80,000 others, Scoutetten lists camp followers at 8,000.[15] Yet, in this climate of conjecture, an order of magnitude is no great matter. Zeros may come or go; there is no basis for complaint other than departure from some equally arbitrary figure. Usually, it was more important that numbers be big than that they be right. Cholera writers wanted the disease to be taken seriously. That uncountable Indians were dying conveyed that message, and another too: don't be black.

These figures could be brandished, and yet readily discarded. Cure rates, for example, were apt to be judged in terms of what was considered possible in the population in question. "If we could have the slightest confidence ... [in Kolkata figures showing a ten percent case mortality rate], we must believe that the disease could be handled far more successfully then, than in modern times," Macpherson concluded. But that was impossible for a true cholera; either the numbers or the diagnoses were wrong.[16]

Minds

The role of mind in cholera was a second site of divisiveness. Both before and after 1817, clinicians would list unease among cholera's symptoms. It might come a few days or a few hours before the vomiting and purging began. Feeling uneasy at breakfast, Munro, governor of Madras, knows he has taken cholera. He is dead in ten hours. This cholera "malaise" might be seen as a partial cause or as an early stage of the disease itself. To some, mental state was the most conspicuous distinction between those who got cholera and those who did not. Officers' relative immunity was partly due to their greater personal autonomy, which reflected "the greater influence of mind, and the amusement which it creates," Orton wrote.[17]

Orton thought he knew how unease related to cholera; the pathology had been elucidated in recent decapitation experiments. For the brief span of remaining vitality, the headless animal subjects had cholera symptoms: they spasmed, their limbs became cold, urine flow ceased, all as in cholera. Analogy was seductive certainly, but surely decapitation was simply the epitome of depression ("you think you're having a bad day..."), which in turn was the essence of cholera.[18]

Most cholera writers would fix on a single species of depressing passion: fear, particularly of cholera. Some choleras ("Angst-Cholera") might be caused entirely by fear. Hence the way *not to get* cholera was not to worry about *getting* cholera. Yet any rational assessment of near-term threats would dictate precisely the opposite: you should be scared; you would not be worrying about cholera unless it was raging all around you...and so on. Yet, as Hawkins puts it, "The imagination should *not be allowed*, for a moment, to dwell on the painful considerations which the disease is calculated to bring before the mind; and least of all ought the dread of it to be encouraged."[19]

Whatever was done, then, must contribute to confidence. If people believed in what doctors and governments were doing to conquer cholera, cholera would be conquered, but whether by that confidence or those acts one could never know. The authorities might feel warranted in denying an epidemic or misdiagnosing an individual case for therapeutic reasons. When cholera hit Murcia in 1885, the local government's "first effort was to infuse heart and courage into the inhabitants by seeking to conceal the real truth," as its representative explained.[20] Or they might invoke quarantine, even for a non-contagious disease, because people believed in it. "The fear of cholera is almost the only predisposing cause in this country [England], which could give strength to the enemy, or prevent...[cholera] from soon expiring by the natural resistance of the climate," declared James Johnson in *The Times*.[21]

Fighting cholera by positive thinking led to ironies, enigmas, paradoxes, and mixed messages. Consider, for example, the advice of the Russian Government in 1830 (advice repeated with little modification by other governments for much of the century). The first seven of twelve items dealt with diet (remember breakfast, avoid fruit), personal hygiene (change linen as often as possible, keep body, house, street clean); clothing (stay warm and change damp socks), and air (ventilate but do not sleep outdoors). The next four explained how to recognize cholera and where to get medical help. Finally, the Czar's ministers addressed the confidence problem:

> The authorities of the government, *founding their confidence on the assurance given them by medical men,* who have carefully attended to the progress of the disorder, inform the citizens *with certainty,* that they will be *preserved from its attacks* if they conform themselves *exactly to the directions* above laid down. A very important means of safety is *to repress* all tendency to depression and chagrin, and to preserve a cheerfulness and tranquility of mind.[22]

The guarantee of safety from cholera is backed by the credit of the medical profession but compromised by the fine print of rule-following, even in the case of rules (like those on hygiene) that are indefinite. But, having asked for a vote of confidence, the final statement undercuts confidence. If we must *also* be cheerful Charlies, how good can the rest of the advice be? Is the government appealing to our rationality or demanding irrationality? And how are we to combine the constant watch for cholera's early rumblings with the devil-may-care tranquility needed to avoid the scourge?

How then to gain (the illusion of) confidence? Again, chiefly by division. For surely there was an elect whom cholera did

TO THE INHABITANTS OF THE PARISH OF

CLERKENWELL.

His Majesty's Privy Council having approved of precautions proposed by the Board of Health in London, on the alarming approach OF THE

INDIAN CHOLERA

It is deemed proper to call the attention of the Inhabitants to some of the Symptoms and Remedies mentioned by them as printed, and now in circulation.

Symptoms of the Disorder;

Giddiness, sickness, nervous agitation, slow pulse, cramp beginning at the fingers and toes and rapidly approaching the trunk, change of colour to a leaden blue, purple, black or brown; the skin dreadfully cold, and often damp, the tongue moist and loaded but flabby and chilly, the voice much affected, and respiration quick and irregular.

REMEDIES:

All means tending to restore circulation and to maintain the warmth of the body should be had recourse to without the least delay.

The patient should be immediately put to bed, wrapped up in hot blankets, and warmth should be sustained by other external applications, such as repeated frictions with flannels and camphorated spirits, poultices of mustard and linseed (equal parts) to the stomach, particularly where pain and vomiting exist, and similar poultices to the feet and legs to restore their warmth. The returning heat of the body may be promoted by bags containing hot salt or bran applied to different parts, and for the same purpose of restoring and sustaining the circulation white wine wey with spice, hot brandy and water, or salvolatile in a dose of a tea spoon full in hot water, frequently repeated; or from 5 to 20 drops of some of the essential oils, as peppermint, cloves or cajeput, in a wine glass of water may be administered with the same view. Where the stomach will bear it, warm broth with spice may be employed. In every severe case or where medical aid is difficult to be obtained, from 20 to 40 drops of laudanum may be given in any of the warm drinks previously recommended.

These simple means are proposed as resources in the incipient stages of the Disease, until Medical aid can be had.

THOS. KEY,
GEO. TINDALL, *Churchwardens.*

Sir GILBERT BLANE, Bart. in a pamphlet written by him on the subject of this Disease, recommends persons to guard against its approach by moderate and temperate living, and to have in readiness the prescribed remedies; and in case of attack to resort thereto immediately but the great preventative he states, is found to consist in a *due regard to Cleanliness and Ventilation.*

N.B. It is particularly requested that this Paper may be preserved, and that the Inmates generally, in the House where it is left may be made acquainted with its contents.

NOV. 1st, 1801.

T. GOODE, PRINTER, CROSS STREET, WILDERNESS ROW.

5. Did notices like this one, referring to the 'alarming approach of Indian cholera' and detailing sure-fire self help remedies to use before medical aid arrived, relieve anxiety or create it? Remarkably, here cholera's symptoms include neither diarrhea nor vomiting. (*Wellcome Library, London*)

not strike. One separated those who would be cholera victims from whatever identity one claimed for oneself, in terms of race, nation, class, constitution, persona, or grace—whatever came to hand. Authors took pains to include among the elect those who might think themselves excluded. Orton's brave officers might keep their heads under cholera's attack, but what about women? Might they, experiencing a slight diarrhea, worry themselves into cholera? Perhaps, another suggested, at least some women excelled in a "moral courage...possessed by individuals who are even the weakest, perhaps, as respects physical powers, and which in them resists more efficiently the causes of intertropical diseases, than the bodily powers of the strongest." To read that such persons existed was an invitation to become one. Hawkins thought doctors gained *moral* protection from cholera by their *knowledge* of the laws of hygiene—separately from their following of those laws.[23] Another counseled moral resistance even after one came down with cholera. It was "surrender to the disease" that made it deadly; "if they kept up courage and fought the disease for an hour or two, and submitted to proper treatment, the chances are in favor of recovery." Some bravehearts were back to work within three hours.[24] A third cholera writer declared that reading his book "*will* have the effect of doing away with one of the most predisposing causes of the susceptibility to attack of most epidemic diseases, viz., Fear." That was all the more likely when the reader—who would, we may presume, be someone with sufficient means to buy cholera books—read statements like the following (from Scoutetten).

- In Europe, the number of upper-class cholera victims had been "extremely small; their names, indeed, might be easily enumerated."

- "When such instances have occurred among the affluent classes, they might probably be explained by particular mental anxiety, or a state of predisposing bad health."
- Cholera "selected such as live in filth and intemperance:...a person of undaunted mind, with cleanliness and moderation was safe from attack."
- "the pusillanimous alone die from...[cholera]."[25]

Drink, dance, and God

As appeals to the power of reading suggest, the distinction between artificially becoming someone whom cholera would pass by and naturally being such a person was narrow and ambiguous. There were other ways to cholera freedom—drink, for example. Hawkins advised doctors to fortify themselves with drink before attending cholera patients: external spirits kept up the internal spirits. Courage need not be well warranted to be strongly felt. While cholera control is frequently associated with temperance, early writers were often ambivalent about alcohol. As Orton pointed out, the problem was not drinking but stopping, coming off a binge into mental and physical depression and the "same extreme anxiety, causeless terror and despondency, which are characteristic of cholera."[26]

The need to deny or distract the mind from incipient cholera may also explain the puzzling phenomenon of cholera balls. Best known is Edgar Allen Poe's "Masque of the Red Death" (1842), often seen as a literary response to the cholera epidemic Poe experienced in Baltimore in 1832. But in Paris too cholera was mocked in balls; and Mary Lennox's parents are partying when cholera strikes them.

If not drink and diversion, then perhaps faith? "The clergymen of the place should continually endeavour to inspire confidence in Divine Providence, and to tranquillize and strengthen the mind." Thus Hawkins advised cholera pep talks; God, like drink, had instrumental value in a pinch. Community services of prayer and penance, fast days in faiths that did not usually fast, would be a feature of early responses to cholera, not just in Europe and America, but in India, China, Japan, and Korea. Writers often urge a private trust in Providence as well. But was this faith or distraction? Hawkins's allusion suggests that he for one would not have gained confidence from the best of sermons. Similarly ambivalent was Rudyard Kipling in "The Cholera Camp" (1896), on an Anglo-Indian regiment steadily losing soldiers as it marches on.

> We've got the cholerer in camp—it's worse than forty fights;
> We're dyin' in the wilderness the same as Isrulites;
> It's before us, an' be'ind us, an' we cannot get away,
> An' the doctor's just reported we've ten more to-day!

But luckily the ranks include parson and padre.

> Our Chaplain's got a banjo, an' a skinny mule 'e rides,
> An' the stuff 'e says an' sings us, Lord, it makes us split our sides!
> With 'is black coat-tails a-bobbin' to *Ta-ra-ra Boom-der-ay!*
> 'E's the proper kind o' *padre* for ten deaths a day.

> An' Father Victor 'elps 'im with our Roman Catholicks —
> He knows an 'eap of Irish songs an' rummy conjurin' tricks;
> An' the two they works together when it comes to play or pray;
> So we keep the ball a-rollin' on ten deaths a day.

But what of the non-cynical faithful? Fear God and there was no need to fear cholera. The epitome of fearlessness as a cholera preventive was placing one's fate in God's hands; cholera would come or not, as God(s) willed. Yet nineteenth-century European cholera writers generally adopt a loosely Christian activism. One prays to God to stay the cholera, but only fools expect prayer to substitute for quarantine, disinfection, or removal of nuisances. In the event of cholera, John Austin tells us "to shew with humble submission to the will of unerring Providence, an undaunted front." This means putting trust both in nature ("our variable climate...herein our friend") and culture: cleanliness, airiness, good food, "domestic comforts," and medical skill. The tone is hardly "humble" or submissive.[27]

To these writers, chief among those fools were Asians, benighted enough to think the God(s) really heard their prayers and that prayer or penance was the most that should be done. They were simply exhibiting so-called oriental fatalism, a misplaced trust in the cosmos to work as it would. Though applied mostly to Islam and to China, the designation could be applied also to Hinduism, since the intercession sought from deities was seen as an alternative to practical means to fight cholera. Besides oversimplifying, the designation had enormous rhetorical utility. Another's suffering, apathy, and hopelessness became philosophic choice or freely chosen faith. The ravages of cholera were expressions of cultural self-determination. Thus wielded, "culture" could explain away state failures, corruption, tyranny, poverty, ignorance, or simply an appalling lack of compassion. Where fatalism prevails, governments can do nothing—should do nothing.

On a global scale, religion was the greatest source of divisiveness. The religious wars are fought anew in the pages of cholera books, for cholera provided an index of God's pleasure and displeasure. Before 1832 some Americans were smug: "The history of cholera seemed to demonstrate that those countries with fewest Christians had been scourged most severely."[28] After it became clear that Christian countries were being hit, and hard, cholera took on sectarian utility as an index of apostasy. To late-nineteenth century Jesuits it marked the failure of scientism; to Italian conservatives the failure of anticlericalism, the Enlightenment, and nationalism together.

But the strongest divisions are between east and west, modern and ancient, reasoned faith and superstition. Ostensible toleration of eastern religions is often belied by coy observations of incidents in which Asian cholera-coping backfires. Thus, the King of Siam, orchestrating a religious festival to forestall cholera in 1820: seven thousand died on the spot. Likewise, the secret ceremonies of the Hajj, particularly the sacrifice of Coram Balram, indicated the insanitary absurdity of Asian religions: tens of thousands would have been "wallowing in the putrefying heaps of blood and offal of victims sacrificed at the feast." (Nelson, the author, then admits that putrefying flesh is not a factor in contagious cholera.) Writing in 1885 of an anti-cholera ceremony that led to all twenty-seven cholera deaths in Foochow, an American diplomat is only slightly more restrained: this

> idolatrous procession...had paraded the streets in the night and rain for the purpose of warding off the disease. Such occasions are always accompanied with much imprudent eating and drinking, thus fitting the participants for an attack and rendering them unable to recover...The parading of the idols...comprise the various sanitary measures employed in Foochow to prevent the ravages of cholera.[29]

When panic and flight followed, Europeans had an occasion to revile the fatalistic faith they had conjured up. The implicit accusation was hypocrisy.

Festivals and pilgrimages were particularly prominent in such renderings. In India, the triennial pilgrimages to Hardwar (Haridwar) would repeatedly be blamed for spreading cholera. Within India, Hardwar came to embody the tension between freedom of religious practice and restrictive health-based government.[30] These great fairs would come to rival the health of the military as the most prominent context of Indian cholera. Similarly, outbreaks among pilgrims in Mecca became a significant source of international tension in the late nineteenth century, as we will see in the next chapter. Such events coalesced with other idioms of divisiveness. Festivals, attracting from tens of thousands to millions, were occasions of fanaticism as of fatalism: here were the anonymous and anarchic Asian masses oblivious to individual life and death. Explorer Baker condemned "holy shrines as the pest spots of the world."[31]

During the last third of the century this revulsion to religious gatherings would be translated into the idiom of the waterborne cholera germ. Christie worried that the water of the holy well of Zem Zem had purgative properties from dissolved salts. Drunk by fatigued travelers, it would predispose to cholera; given the absence of sanitary facilities in Mecca—"the entire surface of the district is covered with dejecta"—that water would be "saturated with the germs of diseases." Hindu rituals, too, were often water centered.[32]

To recognize the manifold utility of "fatalism," however, gets us no closer to the question of how cholera was being assimilated. Teachings were not necessarily lived values. The Anglo-Indian government's strategic decision after 1857, to pursue a policy of cultural non-interference, does allow us sometimes to see that religious expression might well be more important to some Hindus and Muslims than anti-cholera measures.

Concern for comfort and physical safety on a spiritual journey that would manifest trust in God seemed misplaced, if not insulting. Yet the policy—that Indians might die of cholera by the millions if that was the Indian thing to do—has been, understandably, condemned. David Arnold argues that many Indians looked to the British to take much more aggressive actions against pilgrimage-related cholera.

Particularly to liberal Westerners trying to make religious sense of this new scourge, the so-called fatalism of the Orient, and particularly Islam, was genuinely confusing. They came to cholera with an expectation that God intended the world to be changed, not endured. Epidemics, like other aspects of the fallen world, were sent to teach and to prod. As a Congregationalist missionary in the Ottoman Balkans in the middle of the nineteenth century, my great-great-grandfather returned repeatedly to the theme of Islamic fatalism. When his Muslim guide took him across a steep scree slope in Macedonia, Cyrus Hamlin was horrified. If God wanted them to get across, they would, was the reply. When it came to cholera, Hamlin noted, "the Moslems and the Jews were the greatest sufferers; the latter for their filth, the former for their fatalism." He told of a "pleasant old Turkish neighbor," dining on a cucumber. Didn't he know the dangers of raw vegetables, especially cucumbers, during cholera? "'What do I care,' he replied. 'What is written is written...My appetite demands these and I shall eat them.' He died...during the night."[33]

To the activist Hamlin, by inclination more engineer than preacher, this was both admirable and wrong headed. Cholera represented something broken that needed fixing—by medicines in the short term, by sanitation and civilization in the long. He had no medical training, but bodies were not so different from steam engines (he had built the first in Turkey).

Having investigated over a hundred cases, read much, and corresponded with other missionaries, he worked out remedies and took up doctoring. As he explained in his own short cholera treatise (1865): "having been providentially compelled to have a good deal of practical acquaintance with [cholera], and to see it in all its forms and stages…I wish to make my friends in America some suggestions which may relieve anxiety, or be of practical use."[34]

Hamlin's own cholera theology was ambiguous. He attributed most cholera to drink, dietary error, or "suppressed perspiration." True understanding followed by correct action could prevent it most of the time. But the same providence that had put him in the midst of cholera also allowed human error—"thoughtless indiscretions of some member of a household"—which might occasionally bring cholera even into the households of such righteous New Englanders. Luckily, its cure could be accomplished by the priesthood of all believers: intelligent, reasoning, and disciplined persons required no dubious medical intermediary. The right medicines—laudanum, spirits of camphor, and tincture of rhubarb—had to be immediately at hand. (This was "Mixture No. 1"; "Mixture No. 2", of capsicum, cardamom, and ginger was for more serious cases.) Cholera never came without warning and could be prevented or mitigated by decisive action. During an epidemic, one was to be alert to "the slightest variation of feeling," all the while making sure to discard any imaginary feeling. Convinced by diarrhea that fleeting pain or rumbling belly signified something real, one began treatment and kept it up even after the problem seemed to have passed. Think yourself well; believe you have missed the cholera? "You will repent of your folly in vain. I have seen many a one commit suicide in this way," declared preacher Hamlin.[35]

The view of fatal illness as suicide was the antithesis to any fatalism. However much Hamlin admired Turkish courage, he held what would become the main Protestant view of cholera: the product of laws equally natural and providential, it signaled human failure and was a test of the character, here seen as discipline, of individuals and cultures. The metaphors were military: recovery required "perfect rest," no matter how well one felt. To lie absolutely still (resisting any spasms, one assumes) was "half the battle. In that position the enemy fires over you, but the moment you rise you are hit."[36]

"Filth" and loathing

Most important in Hamlin's sweeping declaration about cholera causes is this generalized "filth." Is it filth of person, of household, or of street? He does not say. Generally, in the nineteenth-century sanitary literature, "filth" would require no translation; the value of the term was to package description and evaluation; accusation and conviction; and corrective action into one term. Remarkably, the earlier Anglo-Indian surgeons had not fixed on filth in explaining cholera. James Kennedy (1832) loathed everything about Kolkata, including its poverty. Parts of it were filthy, but that was fact, not moral-visceral response.[37] Filth–disease associations were long-standing; they were linked to no single theory of disease causation. Were these writers too distant from the lives of Indians to notice or care? My sense is that they saw no need to belabor what could only be idle accusation.

It is not until cholera reaches Europe (Russia) that the cholera–filth equation begins to predominate over the cholera–poverty equation. The difference between Hawkins's emphasis on poverty and Scoutetten's filth revulsion, written a few months later, is profound. As he writes, cholera had reached Vienna, and Scoutetten sought to explain why it had been devastating in some places but not others. Poverty was a factor, but barbarism and race (and place) were more important. Cholera singled out "men who indulge in excesses of every kind" and "negroes," among whom "want of cleanliness, and warm temperatures, are among the most active causes." Scoutetten's list of cholera calumnies was a long one. Cholera burst forth in India where parents (in times of famine) sold children, and particularly in Bengal, where they ate (and drank the blood of) dogs, frogs, and serpents, and in Indonesia, where they "smoke opium with tobacco, and when intoxicated, attack the first one they see."

Filth talk represented the poor not simply as suffering from cholera but as responsible for it. Europe suffered according to its geographic and cultural similarity to the East. Cholera was in Hungary because its climate was oriental—that, and because its peasantry were dirty, poorly fed, gave in to excesses, slept on the cold ground rather than in taverns, were shod in rags, sewed themselves into their clothes, and wore greasy hairpieces. Worse were "the [Polish] peasants...perhaps more dirty and more unhappy than in any country of Europe." They lived in damp forests and among stagnant waters, on coarse food and too much brandy. Here, too, there was bad hair: the "men cover their heads with a bonnet of greasy wool which is not moved for whole months." This *plica polonica*—a mode of hairstyling similar to dreadlocks—was, to Scoutetten, "a singular and disgusting disease," but how it figures in cholera he does not say. [38]

Cholera did not follow every route or rage everywhere with equal intensity, Scoutetten could point out only sixteen cases in Odessa, fifteen in Tripoli. For France, the standard response of the *cordon sanitaire* of troops on the border, with orders to shoot trespassing foreign pestilants, would not be needed. In autocratic Russia, cholera exacerbated tensions between rich and poor and between Russians and their imperial subjects, including Jews and Poles. It was all so unlike France, with its "fine climate…habits, manners, the cleanliness of our houses and cites, our modes of living, our food and drink" (and, of course, superior hair dressing). If cholera came to France, it would do little harm. Likewise with Prussia, particularly Berlin and Königsburg, where, one suspects, the shade of Immanuel Kant would simply determine that it was not *Ding an sich*. Scoutetten was an optimist on cholera, but he too believed in the power of positive thinking: compared to the black death, cholera was not so big a deal.

Cholera did not merely reflect the main fault lines of societies; it was a political and sectarian resource. In Scoutetten's France, or England, or America, power was broadly distributed. Axes of opposition were multiple; there was ample occasion to imagine how one's own group was endangered by others. Conflicts having to do with the extension of democracy, the creation of national identity from multiple ethnicities, the rivalry between industry and agriculture, peasant and landlord, proletarian and owner; or between some orthodoxy and multiple heterodoxies or modernist materialism could all be fought with cholera. Immigrants and strangers were a cholera threat; so too were the traditional targets of opprobrium, Jews and gypsies, even into the early twentieth century.

As proxy for cholera and other disease, "filth" was the most common defining element for finger-pointing, a catchall for any species of other. It was less condition than identity. We think of filth in terms of sanitary conditions, but it needed no referent and invited hearers not to expect one. The utterance was distancing enough; no need to make it into a hypothesis subject to empirical test. Rosenberg quotes an assessment of the choleraic apocalypse from an American religious paper in 1832; it is not very different from the assessments of French and Italian bishops writing in the 1880s. *"Drunkards and filthy, wicked people of all descriptions,* are swept away *in heaps,* as if the Holy God could no longer bear their wickedness, just as we sweep away a mass of filth when it has become so corrupt that we cannot bear it."[39] Whether radical (Banim) or conservative, this filth–cleanliness antithesis was far more than epidemiological generalization. Filth marked the reprobate; cleanliness was redemption.

Paranoia runs deep

Did cholera actually single out the vicious? Hardly exclusively. In Russia, a lower middle class of (presumably virtuous) shop-keepers suffered more heavily than the abject peasantry. In America one doctor hid the fact that drunkards seemed peculiarly immune. But often the poor and transient did suffer disproportionately. If so, what story did *they* tell? They do not say, "You are right. I am filthy. Witness my cholera." Filth accusations do not generate filth confessions.

Cholera riots—instances of direct action against the authorities—occurred frequently. How many there were is impossible to know, but no region seems unrepresented, and the resistance continues over a long period. Riots were still occurring in the south of Italy in 1910–11. The riots were not about being despised; usually they were about being murdered. We die because those in power want us dead. "Cholera" is their cover story.

The poisoning accusation appears in cholera's first European stop in Moscow. A correspondent, Christine, claims a wave of arsenic poisonings in July 1831. Convenient "cholera" deaths included a general (Debtisch) who had lost battles. There, cholera-as-poisoning was seen as an expedient mode of personnel change among the powerful as well as a way to cull the poor. Poisoning rumors could consolidate patriotism; the poisoners were surely Polish fifth columnists.

Historians have dismissed such claims, making them a measure of cholera hysteria. Real cholera is not from arsenic; it is the infectious disease of Snow and Koch. But we interpret rather than investigate. That the poor—of Paris, Naples, Moscow, or Manila—*could* believe something so bizarre shows how alienated they had become from legitimate authority.

Among cholera historians François Delaporte pioneered in making credible the view from below. For the "dangerous classes" of Paris, deadly bowel disease was normal.[40] Why, then, the fuss about cholera? Surely because "epidemic" was really genocide—the Malthusian authorities accelerating an inadequate death rate. The fact that cholera struck adults of childbearing age added to the interpretation of genocide; so, too, did the disinfection squads (often armed), who stole or destroyed contaminated household goods, actions which suggested that those they spirited off to isolation wards—victims and exposed others—would not be coming back.

Powerlessness became proof of such speculations. The presence of officialdom was the presence of rule. Rule was the will of the powerful. If cholera coincided with all that, it too was the will of the powerful. Outright resistance might not always be called for, but nor was enthusiastic cooperation or appreciation.

Paris is hardly the only site. Albanesi described Palermo in 1885. There were suddenly "all sorts of regulations and...abundant disinfections." Those "generally neglected and frequently ill-treated" became the target of the "most assiduous care." They saw that cholera coincided with cholera relief: "Unable to discriminate between good and evil...they refused assistance, shut themselves up, barricaded the doors of their houses, and when one offered them any aid, replied, 'Let me die in peace.'"[41] Governments faced a conundrum. The more vigorously they *acted to combat* cholera, the more clearly they declared their responsibility *for cholera*.

Such responses confront historians with a dilemma. We measure the depth of alienation in the height of the irrationality. Snowden writes of a "combustible" mix of illiteracy and distrust, which "degenerated into an atmosphere of hysteria."[42] Sympathy distances us from them, for we occupy the seat of truth on this matter of what "cholera" really was.

Are we so sure they are wrong? In fact, "cholera" as poisoning was a product not of the deranged imaginations of the desperate poor, but of learned medical writers. They agreed (and still agree) that cholera symptoms are difficult to distinguish from those of many organic and inorganic poisons (including, ironically, substances like strychnine or mercury considered as therapeutic agents against cholera). Orton asserted "a strong analogy...between the effects of the poisons and cholera," even "to the extent of perfect identity." He reported cholera-like symptoms from verdigris, mushrooms, snake bites, extracts from several trees from the Malayan archipelago (including that from which strychnine was extracted), and oysters (for us, only the last, contaminated with *Vibrio cholerae*, would be the real thing). He was working on the assumption that like effects had like causes.[43] The great Spanish toxicologist Mateo Orfila worked from the other end of the analogy, comparing an overdose of tartar emetic to *cholera morbus*. Nelson, writing a generation later, saw cholera's suddenness as indicative of toxic action. Affecting all parts at once, cholera was less a disease than a powerful assault on vitality akin to falling from a height or being shot through the heart.[44] And, of course, we currently understand cholera pathology in terms of a local toxin (released by *Vibrio cholerae*).

Pollitzer did work out a differential diagnosis between cholera and food—or mineral—poisonings in the 1950s, based on the timing and character of stools. But an inexperienced (and unsuspicious) clinician might well miss them. "A cholera epidemic," Rosenberg mused, was indeed "an ideal occasion for the removal of unwanted spouses, affluent and immoderately aged uncles, and the like."[45]

Further, if cholera therapies were often themselves poisons, and if the result of their application was often death, it became harder to draw a line between the willful acts of a criminal poisoner and the therapeutic acts of the physician trying harsh treatments in a deadly disease. Yet, while we ridicule dangerous therapies, historians avoid the language of poisoning. Intent makes all the difference.

Too simple? Physicians had many roles in cholera epidemics: to heal, to sequester transients or to incarcerate victims, to learn, and to teach. Hospitalization was undertaken to isolate the contagious as well as to cure (some Parisians wondered why removal was so important if cholera required prompt action). Efforts to learn from dissection could be read as orchestrated killing to get cadavers.

In light of the frequent futility of conventional means, the most altruistic physicians might be attracted to an experimental medicine of "great and desperate" cures. In Naples, in 1884, a gulf existed between established practitioners who trusted opium, calomel, and superior clinical skill to save some, and younger doctors who saw that as irresponsible complacency. Better to try more aggressive treatments, such as electro-shock therapy, or irrigation of the ileum by germ-killing carbolic acid (administered, sometimes, with the patient inverted, via an enema strong enough to push past the check valve that normally kept matters from returning from the large to the small bowel). Failure in novel treatments was not necessarily reason for their rejection. Ingredients, doses, timings, and modes of administration might be varied; the physician's duty was to keep trying and learning. Informed consent was far in the future; those on whom the remedies were tried—the forcibly hospitalized poor—did not get to choose. Well into the twentieth century, cholera remained the site of enormous and unregulated experiments.

Poisoning is an ugly word, but medical intervention probably did contribute to many cholera deaths. Hardly surprising, then, that rioters often targeted doctors and hospitals. Disproportionately suffering from cholera, Scoutetten's Hungarian shepherds concluded that doctors and nobles had conspired "to poison them…[which] caused them to revolt and massacre those brave men, who had faced death to save them." Applying "physician, heal thyself" to epidemiological reasoning, some Russian villagers abducted two doctors trying to enforce a household quarantine, bound them to cholera corpses, and threw them into a pit. If they survived, they would be able to testify that cholera was not contagious. (They were pulled out and lived.)[46]

However apolitical they might think themselves, doctors did not practice outside political contexts. When French doctors gave shock treatments to Italian guest workers, their patients inferred murderous intent. French patients got the same treatment, but the Italians felt unwelcome in France. Quasi-Malthusian (or later social Darwinist) currents were rarely very far below the surface. Certainly there was no reason to think per se that the unfamiliar state doctor was one's friend.

And it was not just doctors. When they distributed free food and medicine to the cholera stricken in mid 1880s Sicily, even the priests were

> hooted at and insulted, [even] with the bishop of the diocese at the head. It was found impossible to induce the people to make use of medicines distributed without some person of the local committee acting the part of taster...and even then, when the course of the disease was rapid and fatal, the symptoms were frequently attributed to the medicine administered, rather than to the disease.[47]

Generally cholera recovery rates fell during the second half of the nineteenth century (probably from more restrictive diagnosis). A recovery rate of 50 percent was about the best to be hoped for. Under such circumstances, the request to be let to "die in peace" was not an unreasonable one.

Except during brief spans—for example, Italy at the time of the Borgias or the Rome of Agrippina and Nero—historians have not imagined a past full of poisoning. Our neglect is caution: what is not documented cannot be said to have happened. Yet, *accusation* of cholera as poisoning *is* widespread; still we simply smile at the claims. Were we to enlarge the concept to include slowly as well as rapidly acting agents; omission as well as commission; carcinogens, mutagens, and endocrine disrupters, and microbial and viral agents, then the perspective shifts. As we wonder why preventable deaths are not prevented, we can readily think ourselves into the logic of Delaporte's Parisians or Albanesi's Palermitans. At issue is culpability. Cholera, says one of Charles Kingsley's characters, is always "someone's fault: and if deaths occur, someone ought to be tried for manslaughter—I had almost said for murder."

Kingsley, Osborne: cholera as the fall of all

In an odd way, cholera riots were a part of a liberalizing agenda. As Albanesi recognized, they reflected a violation of implicit contracts and of customs. They disclosed gaps between the promise of progress and its delivery. Often the paranoia had foundation. After 1830 "cholera" had been transformed from an innocuous disease of anybody into an index of guilt—by race, class, or sometimes confession. Even if it did not enhance conflict along these divisions, cholera offered a way to explain and justify it.

But, beginning around 1850, partially, incompletely, and ever so slowly, cholera would begin to shift back to being a problem of all. God was not smiting some, but making clear how all must live. Long ago, Rosenberg documented this change in America, where it was reasonably complete by the mid 1860s. It occurred in Britain about the same time, reflecting a common liberal Protestantism. Yet it was not quickly applied to colonial populations, nor, as Briggs and Martini-Briggs have ably shown, is it complete in the twenty-first century. Better knowledge contributed, but that shift was not mainly scientific. Rather it was an ethical and prophetic shift, one not merely reflected in religious interpretations of cholera, but essentially a theological shift, reflecting a revolution in theodicy. Put simply, cholera ceased to signify sins that some committed or inexplicable divine will, and began to be seen in terms of original sin, an unfortunate (and redeemable) aspect of the normal workings of nature.

Here the exemplar is the mid-nineteenth-century Anglican clergyman Charles Kingsley (1809–75), known as one of the earliest clerical champions of Darwin and author of *The Water Babies*. Kingsley confronted cholera as preacher and apologist; as pastor and community leader; as novelist, essayist, and inspirational speaker. He was almost a cholera researcher; his Christian socialist colleague (and his wife's brother-in-law), Reverend Lord Sidney Godolphin Osborne (1809–89), was, in a minor way.

Cholera struck England in 1848–9 and again in 1853–4, the richest years of Kingsley's career. Responding to incipient revolution in spring 1848, he and some friends founded the Christian Socialist movement. They accepted that there was warrant for revolution. If the souls (and bodies) of London slum-dwellers could not flourish, government had failed. As cholera threatened, they began a campaign of sanitary relief, carting water to the east London neighborhood of Jacob's Island, whose residents had relied on an ancient sewer-ditch.

In three successive weeks in September 1849, Kingsley explained cholera to his country parishioners in the Hampshire village of Eversley. There he attacked the public prayers and penitential services, days of fast, and quick dose of good works that had been the typical religious response to cholera. Penitence was in order, but it had to be directed to the sins that had brought on the cholera. Kingsley's was not a kinder, gentler God and certainly not a patient one. He worked by natural laws. "God's judgment" manifest in cholera was failure to learn cholera science; redemption was research and then prevention. "God punishes…not by His caprice, but by His laws. He does not *break His laws* to harm us; the laws themselves harm us, when we break them."[48] Those laws operated at the level of societies not individuals. Plainly, cholera also killed the innocent, the clean, and children.

That unasked-for sociality was none other than the concept of original sin, which, for Kingsley, was less a mark of innate wickedness than a sign of universality. Cholera's transmissibility was another indication of that inescapable sociality: "God made of one blood all nations...The same food will feed us all alike. The same cholera will kill us all alike."[49] But, being wholly preventable, cholera was a fate freely chosen. Thundered Kingsley: "we deserve" the disease we get; epidemics "repeat...by the necessary laws of nature."[50]

All this could be fixed worldwide through a sanitary imperialism (under sanitary English rule). Paraguay had the misfortune to have been colonized by Iberian Catholics, noted Kingsley in 1856: *they* tolerated cholera in their capital cities. Once the Russian steppes were as well tilled "as England is, locusts will be...unknown...Man has no right to have...pestilences [including cholera]...because they can be kept out and destroyed."[51]

The stakes are most fully developed in the best of the cholera novels, *Two Years Ago* (1856), a romance of materialist surgeon Tom Thurnall and Methodist schoolmistress Grace Harvey, set in Aberalva, a fictional north Devon fishing village where Thurnall has, quite literally, washed up (from a shipwreck) just before the 1854 cholera. Thurnall, having fought cholera the world over, can see the epidemic coming, but finds that three factors prevent the village from responding effectively. First is an "I'm alright Jack" attitude: acknowledgment of an insanitary condition requires confession and contrition, an unpleasant introspection. One must say:

> I have been a very nasty, dirty fellow. I have lived contented
> in evil smells, till I care for them no more than my pig does. I
> have refused to understand nature's broadest hints, that any-
> thing which is so disagreeable is not meant to be left about. I
> have probably been more or less the cause of half my own ill-
> nesses, and of three-fourths of the illnesses of my children.

Most will defend their dignity by denial: "sanitary reform is thrust out of sight…too humiliating to the pride of all, too frightful to the consciences of many."

Second is laziness, presenting as fatalism. There are steps to avoid or mitigate cholera, but that requires great energy. They will disrupt roles, rights, and relationships, and probably not work. Heale, the local doctor whose assistant Tom becomes, worries about offending his patients, "if I go a routing and rookling in their drains," and about the expense of nuisances removal. He sees "this new-fangled sanitary reform…[as] a dodge for a lot of young Government puppies to fill their pockets, and rule and ride over us" and finally arrives at the unanswerable assertion that "'tis jidgment, sir, a jidgment of God, and we can't escape His holy will, and that's the plain truth of it." Heale can cite a small catalogue of Old Testament plagues; God sends or lifts them; we can but wait and hope.

Mixed with the laziness was opportunism. A landlord sees the coming of cholera as an opportunity to rid his estate of pauper tenants. Often the opportunism is religious. Sectarians use cholera as an opportunity to attack the Germanizing Anglicanism of preachers like Kingsley himself, who will "explain away the Lord's visitation into a carnal matter of drains, and pipes, and gases, and such like." The saintly Grace is only converted to cholera activism when she realizes that cholera denies its victims a chance to repent. Bodies don't matter, souls do.

Effective response to cholera required more meaning, not less. Grace's (or Kingsley's) activism did not depend on the secularization of cholera, the translating of it into a technical problem, but rather on its translation into religious language and practice. Here fear remained a key element. Thurnall's lectures on the water supply (illustrated with slides of microbe life) "frighten all the children into fits." Both Thurnall and his sectarian adversary recognize that the horrors of cholera rival the horror of hell, and equally that the line between a fear that animates and one that prostrates is thin. Fear of cholera, Kingsley hopes, will spur investment in science and good government that will prevent it, and do much more.

Kingsley shared these themes with his friend Osborne. The aristocratic Osborne had wanted to be a doctor; family pressure had led him into the Church. As SGO (Sydney Godolphin Osborne), he would author a long series of letters to *The Times* on social conditions.

Osborne went further than Kingsley in treating cholera in terms of original sin and redemption. In September 1853, as cholera was returning, he wrote that "bodies reared in filth— souls reared in the midst of blasphemy…men, women, and children who were born amidst filth of body and taint of every moral sense" might still be redeemed. The struggle for them was with cholera: "cholera is taking them, struggling with us for their possession…from amid the filth of physical and moral life cholera grasps them."[52]

In 1854, and again in 1865–6, Osborne sought to translate that struggle into scientific terms: he looked for the germ that might be spread through the environment and cause disease. In 1854 he was looking in the air, using techniques similar to those used by bacteriologists three decades later. Over the top of a cesspool airshaft he placed a glass plate coated with gelatine, and then compared the forms of microscopic life it collected with those normally found in air. He did not find any clear differences, but thought it likely that microbes contributed to cholera. He, like Kingsley, saw benefit in public microscopy: "if the public could be brought to *see* that which floats in what they *smell* from sewers and cesspools, they would be far more careful in the removal of filth…"

In September 1866 he reflected on the increasing evidence that cholera was waterborne, and that even boiling the water might not make it safe. But for Osborne, the whole context for thinking about cholera germs was a providential natural order. Evidently, the world was full of germs: "they may be very poisonous, or may have their part in the economy of health." Perhaps ordinarily benign microbes periodically acquired virulence. Such matters were considered in terms of natural theology, which sounds to us like ecology: "The whole universe is as much, to me, a system of adjustment as is the system of daily life of every animal and vegetable within it. All such systems have been ever subject to more or less disturbance". Was cholera one such disturbance?[53]

Who am I that cholera should come?

The answer to that question was changing; Osborne and Kingsley are pioneers of a coming pattern; their time and place mark a tipping point. None of us is a teeming mass, existing only to be swept away by a deserved scourge. Cholera will become accident, not just desert. If we still recognize and are repelled by certain forms of dirt, our repulsion—I think—does not usually take the form of making that filth the core identity of someone irredeemably "other." We live, after all, in a world of "make-overs"; and there are shovels and soap.

This perspective is common in modern public health. Kingsley and Osborne take a broad ecological view of the relation of humans to infectious diseases. These arise from modes of interaction between human and natural communities, modes that happen to be pathological for some humans. Often, pathogenic interactions are unevenly distributed within communities, yet they have more to do with where and how people are living than with who those people are. And such diseases are still effectively communal; no one in a community experiencing cholera is truly safe.

This sounds like the conclusion of an induction. After 1832 it was plain that Scoutetten had been wrong. Cholera did come to Paris and it killed the brave as well as the fearful, light-skinned people as well as dark-skinned people, and even the rich and well groomed. Yet the change is not from religion to science; from cholera as divine punishment to cholera as natural event; from meanings to facts.

Older views of cholera too had recognized it as a natural phenomenon with natural causes and remedies. One may say they were too naturalistic, too deterministic. The confidence that the liberal Scoutetten can muster depends on an essentially *natural* opposition between Poland and France, and between Polish people and French people, not because of God's love of Frenchmen and hatred of Poles. His assessment rests on a long tradition that is Galenic, neo-Hippocratic, and more immediately filtered through the environmental determinists of the Enlightenment. In such a "constitutional" medicine, it is often noted, cases of disease in individual bodies are overdetermined. The belief that one has given sufficient cause such that the disease in a particular body could not have been anything other than what it was makes disease into a major element of identity and, by one remove, a sign of the diseased one's sin or sad fate. If cholera always knew its victim, one's fate was sealed, and so was the justness of that fate, since nature was simply the executive arm of a God who judged each. Hence the tone of so much of the cholera literature of the 1830s and 1840s: "who am I (or who can I pretend to be) such that cholera will not strike me?" Such a view may invite apathy; if it invites action, that action will be an attempt to alter one's own cosmic status. One may save oneself, but the perspective does not encourage a "public" health.

Kingsley's assignment of cholera to the domain of original sin on the grounds that it kills blameless people is equally a recognition of a phenomenon that is stochastic rather than determinate. All are vulnerable; moreover, given the positive feedback of epidemic disease—that is, that we all become *more vulnerable* the more cholera there is—there is greater emphasis of the dependence of all upon each. Science and religion remain entangled. A larger foundation of empirical knowledge is translated into conceptions of divine action; from these is extracted a broadly applicable generalization of moral philosophy—the principle of human universality with regard to laws of nature, including laws of disease causation—which, when placed in a prophetic framework, warrants a verdict of cholera as unacceptable anywhere and to anyone. In short, cholera becomes both public and publicly problematic.

It did not do so at once, or everywhere, or unambiguously. This new view of cholera did not quickly drive out the old. In Kingsley's own writings, racism often trumps universalism. Nor were the two views as conceptually distinct as they may seem. The eugenic distinction between nature and nurture, heredity and environment, which enacts that same divide, was conspicuous for regular violation of the categories: environment affected hereditary identity, which transformed environment.

The new approach underwrote moral imperialism. Other places and practices had to be transformed to be made safe from cholera; sanitation, broadly conceived, would do that. To late-nineteenth-century Britons, the sanitary mission was pre-eminently British, a project of Europe or civilization only inso-far as it had first been British. But, if the universality of cholera might provide a warrant for a public-health-based imperialism, imperialist practice often shifted back into what I earlier called "withering othering": the representation of filth as freely chosen culture, and of the "natives" as irredeemably other. That perspec-tive, which, some have claimed, held sway in imperial India (and in the American administration of the Philippines), reinforced an ambivalence toward cholera prevention; that is, that it should not be tried because it cannot succeed, because cholera is a mat-ter of something akin to lifestyle if not indeed skin color. If clear in principle, the distinction between "filth" as unanswerable accusation and "filth" as description, diagnosis, even emblem of underdevelopment, unrealized autonomy, and failed delivery of rights, was and is hard to maintain in practice.

Sanitation was also not conspicuously successful as an impe-rial mission, because, for reasons both technical and cultural, it remained at the outer limits of the reach of public policy. It would be local meanings that would be important. If it was a global disease, cholera was almost always experienced locally— it was a matter for those in each place to deal with as well as they could. How well cholera would be controlled depended on what happened in cities, towns, and villages, like Kingsley's Aberalva. A principle of universality did not automatically prevail. A con-cept of cholera citizenship, involving both the right to be free of the disease and the responsibility to help to free one's neighbors from it, had to be conceived, articulated, implemented, learned, instantiated in the built environment, and reproduced generation after generation. No mean feat.

The more we look at such communities, the more we can appreciate how difficult success was, and admire, equally, the bold leadership, trust, courage, hope, persevering work, and effective communal process that an effective response required. Successful responses would require finding ways of uniting disparate groups, mitigating conflict, and minimizing at least some elements of social separation. Could leader-citizens somehow acknowledge paralyzing fear, pervasive terror, and the demand that the disease have meaning without, on the one hand, inviting xenophobia and hysteria or, on the other, giving in to the anodyne of apathy? Could the turmoil that cholera brought actually be directed to dealing with cholera—diverted from settling old scores, confirming tired truths, or furthering ancillary agendas? Must recognition of cholera's sociological distinctiveness—its predilection for the poor—always bring a distancing and dehumanizing of victims? So often efforts to unite were partial; they brought together one segment of a community by isolating it from others. Activism could be seen to—and probably often did—exacerbate both disease and fragmentation.

Many communities in the developed world were sanitized grudgingly and belatedly, in a process of keeping up with legal imperatives or of trying to avoid appearing appallingly backward. Yet for others, there are tipping points, matters jointly technical, environmental, financial, administrative, political, social, and cultural, that embody the phenomenon of path dependence (positive or negative) elucidated by Martin Melosi, and that lead down one road or another, toward cholera or away from it.[54]

III

<del>∞</del>

CITIZEN CHOLERA

"To every thoughtful Physician, such a Visitation as a Cholera Epidemic brings a torrent of deep questionings…[Being] forced to confront…the moral and physical evils which engender or increase Epidemic diseases in our Towns, [one] is to be led into stern communings concerning the whole of our social and political life." So wrote Henry Wentworth Acland, Oxford don and cholera doctor, in the aftermath of the 1854 cholera. A modern historian, Roderick McGrew, notes that "cholera moved like the conscience of the nineteenth century…It settled in the discreetly veiled cesspools of human misery, and it was difficult to ignore the noxious horrors that its presence brought to view."[1] Cholera *made people care*, or so it is claimed.

How hard is it to solve this problem of cholera? From the standpoint of western Europe and North America, it seems easy. Public and government care. Cholera is recognized as a threat to all, and commands resources. The second half of the nineteenth century was the golden age of cholera incidence but also of cholera response—it is often seen as the birth time of modern public health.

In most places cholera returned about once a decade after the 1830s. While the demarcation of distinct pandemics may reveal more about the pandemic-mongers than about epidemics, what is often called the third pandemic of the 1850s was probably the deadliest. One begins to see limited success in prevention/mitigation by the fourth pandemic (the 1860s), in the beginnings of systematic improvement of water and sanitation as well as the exploration of means for sequestering travelers. During the fifth pandemic (the 1880s) Robert Koch's team isolated the cholera vibrio. That discovery had little practical effect: cholera recrossed the world in the first decades of the twentieth century. But it was not stopping everywhere. Britain, as the British repeatedly pointed out, had not had an epidemic since 1866 (despite its connection to cholera-ridden India); other parts of northern and western Europe and North America saw their last epidemics by 1900. Cholera returned to Italy in 1910, and was in Russia in the terrible early 1920s. In India, cholera persisted, following its own rhythms. India was still seen as generator of these waves of cholera, if often on slight evidence. Suspicion that cholera might be transmitted by asymptomatic carriers made it ever harder to challenge such allegations. Whatever ethos of universality had been established rarely extended to Asia.

Political theory in a fecal–oral community

One may ask, "What's conscience to cholera or cholera to conscience?" A common view has cholera doing its own universalizing. Both the disease and the costs and chaos it left affected all. That truth might be denied, but only for a while: the disease was communicable; the cholera of one might become the cholera of any and of all. Hence cholera brought conscience, as we learned to read in another's cholera our own vulnerability.

Britain's experience with cholera and "reform" is often the historical exemplar of this process: efforts in the first third of the nineteenth century to expand political representation called attention to the new industrial towns, home both to the unenfranchised middle classes and to an increasingly desperate casual labor force. Both groups suffered from cholera. As the former gained power after 1832, they worried about the latter as an impediment to stability and prosperity, a problem exacerbated by cholera. These bourgeois would discover in the pipe-bound sanitary city the key to transforming the underclass into citizens, establish a competent and comprehensive state medical bureaucracy to oversee that citizenship, and vanquish cholera in the process. Like all serious problems, cholera would yield to the demand for public accountability; thus public-health achievement is made wholly congruent with human rights and universal compassion (McGrew's "conscience"). Acland sums things up: "to enumerate the arrangements which a wise Community would adopt beforehand to mitigate the terrible scourge of coming Epidemics, is to describe the manner in which a civilized and well-regulated people, acquainted with the laws of health and the causes of disease, would strive to live on ordinary occasions."[2]

The view accounts, I think, for the common assumption that control of cholera will come with democratization, which in turn brings accountability. Together these, with prosperity, constitute some nebulous "development." It also explains the bewildered impatience commonly associated with "failure" to control cholera: "we did it"; "you just do it." Never mind that the scenario does not quite fit for Britain, fits even less well for other places, and rests on dubious assumptions about the inherent character of democracy or the innate power of "conscience."

This chapter explores those assumptions in terms of the strengths and weaknesses of various modes of cholera response. By the beginning of the twentieth century, cholera, by this time largely avoidable, would signify a failure of liberality and modernity, one so flagrant that in 1911 the Italian authorities from the prime minister down would conspire to deny the epidemic. To admit it would invite quarantine, halting trade, blocking necessary emigration, killing tourism. It would equally proclaim how little had changed in a half century of nationalism and republicanism, the incompetence of Italian professionals, the corruption of the state, and the chaos of Italian "democracy." The logic: since the liberal state cannot countenance the cholera, there cannot be cholera. Frank Snowden, uncoverer of the cover-up, protests on behalf of the Italian citizenry and the world community. The needs of citizens could not have been met while their problem was being denied; dishonesty to the world community threatened others who had the right to know. Yet Italy was hardly unique. It was following a pattern set by France and Spain, and by British ship captains.

Cholera denial is alive and well. International health authorities reject quarantine; it is hoped that fostering a guilt-free atmosphere will encourage admission and allow effective response. Yet nations admitting cholera invariably face unwarranted and often long-lasting retribution. Denial makes sense. Italy's denial of cholera was a work of democracy. Prime Minister Giolitti shrewdly saw that maintaining liberal power required writing off the poor of the south; the property and port interests in Naples would not brook interference with their trade. Opponents of the deception—like the embittered

Vatican—were hardly champions of transparency or democracy. In fact, carping was minimal; the deception was not only a rational response but a successful one. Trade was maintained. "Reasons of cholera," like "reasons of state" more broadly, have no necessary connection to the liberal value of transparency or necessary link to liberalism at all.

Moreover, even if there were recognition of the seriousness of the problem and a motivation to solve it, it did not follow that *effective cholera policies* would arise through the legislative arts. Traditionally, aggressive responses to epidemics had involved suppression of liberties (and even the sacrifice of those cordoned off). In the new liberal republics, intelligent policies were to descend from debates and votes in legislatures, no longer from the autocrat's pen. Yet the republics were composites; as in Italy, they were riven by region, religion, ethnicity, class, and ideology. Stability was not the rule, and public action was often paralyzed by conflict. What any single group might hope for was unlikely to be the common weal as conceived by the enlightened autocrats of the late eighteenth century.

Even when legislatures were functional, cholera would not automatically top the list of priorities. Even well-thought-out policies might be stripped of essential features in the market of legislative horse-trading. Getting cholera might be in no one's interest, but particular actions against it were hardly free from sectoral interests. As Acland put it, "the public opinion, which rules in a constitution such as ours, must be frequently in error; and the greater good must for a time too often yield to the less." Policies produced by many minds were not necessarily better than those from one, and often they were worse.

Even were the perfect Platonic cholera policy to fall from the legislative skies, it would still have to be implemented by functionaries who were often ignorant, underpaid, or corrupt—a far cry from the guardians of Plato's republic. Again Acland, complaining of liberal England's failure to have learned from two deadly epidemics: "Though scientific men, aided by the press, have for many years striven to rouse us to a sense of insecurity, the habits of our country, the lengthy labour of discussion which is to be gone through in most public questions, and the precarious results of the votes in public assemblies, retard improvement, and too often ensure mischief."[3]

Complementing the legislature as a liberal institution was the market—public good defined as the composite of the preferences free citizens. How the vector sum of the unfettered operation of social atoms was to deliver health was never clear. Vaccination, for example, was (and is) a conspicuous site of *resistance* to the public good, in the name of liberty. The great liberal theorist John Stuart Mill found it necessary to recognize a residual domain for goods and bads that could not be left to individual choosers. It included matters like sanitation. Charles Kingsley went further: cholera control was the antithesis of laissez-faire. To assert, with the political economists, "There are laws of nature concerning economy, therefore you must leave them alone to do what they like with you and society!" was tantamount to saying: "You got the cholera by laws of nature, therefore you must submit to cholera."[4]

In Kingsley's view people had to be cajoled or bludgeoned into health. "Can it possibly be," mused his friend Acland, "that true social progress and the wisdom of self-government are hardly compatible?"[5] Perhaps not, but "conscience" turns out to be a misnomer. Having acknowledged enlarged rights of their republican citizen-legislators, states expected stability and prosperity from them. But could they deliver all that and cholera control too? Equality, and with it concern for another's cholera or potential cholera, came only after promulgation of an exacting sanitary accountability that was hardly liberal. Along with political citizenship, new terms of "sanitary citizenship" were being forged and tested. This sanitary citizenship was less a matter of moral philosophy—"I would not want this to happen to me, therefore it should not happen to you"—than epidemiology: "knowing where you've come from, I can see that you are safe. We can have relations (or, more graphically, 'I now know that swallowing your excrement will not kill me')." Hence it was not the disease's presence alone but the fact that its control involved *everybody* as potential carrier-victim that explains how it became, for a time, so hard to ignore the "cesspools of human misery."

Perhaps legislatures and markets did not control cholera, yet it was controlled in Europe and America. Puzzling over the modern mortality decline, the epidemiologist Thomas McKeown hypothesized that a rising standard of living was more important than overtly medical solutions for dealing with diseases, even infectious diseases. If McKeown is right, democracy was only a proxy for prosperity. Italy's problem in 1911 was underdevelopment, and only secondarily uneven democratization.

Money is certainly vital to cholera control. Yet macroscopic models like McKeown's take us away from multiple sites where choices were being made about how to spend it. A premise of McKeown's 'rising-tide-floats-all-boats' thesis is that hulls are sound and crews competent, that humans procure the right tools and work well together. We cannot expect that. For most of the nineteenth century the technical problems of cholera were unsolved—there was no cure, no sure means to prevent. Most experimental approaches failed; successes, like providing a community with unimpeachable water, were often partial and transitory, the end of a confusing, lengthy, extraordinarily expensive, and divisive process that strained relationships as it established new forms of authority and, perhaps, new relations of trust, which would constitute the "social capital" in a fecal–oral community.

Acland held that "the largest part of the misery among men depends at last, on moral, not on material causes!"[6] But it is easy to romanticize "social capital" and "community." We should not presume that authority was generally founded on the free gift of citizen trust, or that it bore the hallmark of rationality: a free agent ceding to an expert authority in some well-defined sphere. Custom or peer pressure were often stronger than any measures of performance. Acland's "moral" factors were as subject to failure as the rest.

Unity, prioritization, orderly process, trust and leadership, competence, money: much must go right. One may admit that the best is the enemy of the good, but on matters like cholera it is not clear why we should expect democratic processes or markets to produce even the good. Often they did not and do not.

Accordingly, cholera citizenship is an important issue in nineteenth-century cholera tracts. Cholera was *a res publica* on three levels—first, for states (and for their armies and economies), second for local communities, and third for the community of nations. In the 1830s, states had seemed the natural units of cholera response. While they gradually established effective public-health policies that facilitated the fight against cholera, they failed to stop it in the short term. Cholera challenged myths of command and control; the states' failures put the onus on local governments. Technological changes, chiefly the steam engine, which allowed the rapid transmission of cholera from continent to continent, were a key impetus for rising international concern after 1860. So too were geopolitical factors: Britain was seen to be ruling cholera-ridden India in cavalier fashion, oblivious to the health of the rest.

These levels are more than matters of scale. Cholera's impact was different at each; so too, the schedule, the actors, and the impediments to action were distinct. At each, cholera was an interruption. Societies were not geared for cholera, yet must somehow adapt. Yet adaptation was also opportunity. Careers could be made, ambitions pursued, roles reinforced, goods sold, all the while that cholera was being coped with.

Do that government thing you do

For the government of a state, the most important thing to do in the face of cholera was to *be seen to* be doing something, to be implementing some policy in which hope could be invested. Leadership proved legitimacy; authority required acting authoritatively. The precise action taken mattered less and its success almost not at all. By contrast, to wait to act until one knew the right action might be read as incompetence, irresolution, or even apathy. Only by late in the century would the apparent inaction of ongoing research come to be seen as an adequate response, a matter for the next chapter.

In 1948 the eminent medical historian Erwin Ackerknecht noted that two distinct styles of government response to epidemics, grounded in antithetical theories, prevailed during the years 1821 to 1867. Absolutist states such as Russia, Prussia, and Austria conceived of epidemic disease as an invasion of contagious enemy agents who, having gained a foothold, would pervert the state's subjects to their own ends. Their response was to tighten the borders against potentially contagious persons and things, but also to clamp down on the minimal freedoms they allowed, of movement, assembly, choice of medical care, and religious consolation. That way disease could be locked up. In liberal states, like Britain and France, anticontagionism held sway. Epidemics were transitory states of atmosphere, local, global, or both, which intersected with states of society. Cleaning and strengthening the population might help, but repression gained nothing. Halting trade simply harmed those in vulnerable positions—like the dock worker whose daily wages translated into physiological resistance to the epidemic.

Here I focus on the political side of Ackerknecht's thesis, leaving theory for the next chapter. In broadest terms, the thesis has held up. It works less well for cholera. There it explains initial tendencies, but not persistent policies. It overlooks vacillation. It also oversimplifies and misrepresents the problem cholera posed. Theory did not translate to practice in any unambiguous way. Efforts to prevent contagion by quarantine were not inherently anti-commercial; in the Mediterranean they were more likely to be seen as intrinsic to a well-regulated system of commerce in which trading partners could be confident in the safety of trade. The very assumption of a descent from ideology to practice via theory fixes what was often fluid, and reconstructs a cholera policy that would have made sense had principles been clearly articulated. Yet cholera was not merely a technical problem. It was a problem of institutional ambiguity. Whose job was it to fight cholera? It was a political problem of calibrating expectations to performances. No approach to cholera control was a signal success; it was not clear how much could be hoped for.

These issues were particularly acute in the Russian response. Russia was first of the European states to face cholera. When, in 1829, cholera crossed the frontier near the Caspian Sea, moving up the Volga to Orenburg, Czar Nicholas did what Czars do. Following the precedent of Canute, he ordered it to stop and sent out the army. The army found no identifiable enemy. Cholera arose suddenly in ordinary communities, though these communities were packed with suspicious and uncooperative people (among them, those in charge of local governments). Something must be suppressed, but what? If ordinary doings produced cholera, the people must not do them. They must be kept from fleeing, plucked from the streets, their goods impounded, their bowels sniffed. Through the next two years, as cholera invaded Moscow twice and St Petersburg once, the Army kept up such measures.

They did not work. The Czar did what commanders do next, ordering into action other arms of the autocracy, the doctors and bureaucrats. These could be dispatched from the center, but the model of command and control impeded lateral coordination between branches or the exercise of discretion. Nicholas himself went to the front lines in Moscow—sometimes extraordinary puissance must be enacted directly. He ordered a redoubling of vigilance: increased rigidity of the cordons, the hauling of ever more people off the streets for ever more arbitrary reasons. But there were many front lines of cholera. To command was not to effect.

The Russian government acted as *force majeure* because that was its style. Government was power. Flexibility and creativity, sensitivity to custom and person, the reconciliation of many sectors: none of these was its strong suit.

The problem, there and elsewhere, was threefold. First was the assumption that the cholera problem was one of policy, that one disciplined an unruly world by edicts. Second, assuming the edicts to be warranted (and often they were) was the problem of human imperfection, the slippage between all-wise Czar and executing minion far down the line. Third was the subtlety of cholera itself. It moved faster than the troops, by media hidden to them; sometimes it even moved in them.

There were roughly 400,000 cases and about 190,000 cholera deaths in Russia in 1830–1. McGrew does not mince words: "On balance, the cholera period presented a massive indictment of the autocratic system, of the social and economic foundations on which it rested, and of the men standing at its head." He characterizes the Czar's response as "ignorant despotism": the "blind assault upon the disease with weapons unfitted to the task, blunted by ignorance, and dangerous mainly to their wielders...an open invitation to disaster."[7] And yet, we are told, the Czar's ministrations during the epidemic were widely appreciated; despite the heavier hand, class-based hostility was lower in Russia than in France. Poisoning rumors were not class-specific, as they usually were elsewhere; curiously, the most prominent riots were in St Petersburg, the most westernized part of the empire. Perhaps Russia even succeeded: Moscow's per capita cholera mortality was lower than that of Paris, noted the mid-nineteenth-century Canadian contagionist Robert Nelson; surely that was due to "the strict military discipline and quarantine, and to the closure of infected houses and places."[8] (Others would praise Moscow's open plan and comparatively low housing density.)

Prussia might also have been expected to respond with armies and edicts, but more efficiently, its military having been honed in selective fires since Frederick the Great. It too began with cordons. They were perhaps too efficient, as indicated in the breakdown of authority in the port cities of Danzig and, particularly, Königsburg. There cordons raised food prices. An anti-doctor riot began when a plasterer swallowed acid prescribed for external use, and was fed by disruption of burial customs. Order was only re-established when a force of students and civil servants led by the university's rector (Kant's successor) fired on the crowd, killing seven (cholera had no time for "Enlightenment"). Once breached, cordons had no power against cholera. Prussia lifted them quickly. But, as the Königsburg riots indicated, government itself was in jeopardy.

Britain's response was more farce than deadly drama. Britain got conflicting advice from the expert advisory bodies it established. It made a gesture at quarantine. Then, having authorized local boards of health to deal with the epidemic, the government discovered that these could not legally levy funds and found itself advising citizens to ignore them. In France, notwithstanding an 1822 law permitting cordon-crossers to be shot on sight, Paris was infected in March 1832, probably from multiple directions.

For the next quarter century all these nations would abandon their traditional response of border protection. Regimes used to command would learn to cajole their subject-citizens to keep clean, sober, dry, and well fed, to cooperate with inspectors, and to follow doctors' advice (surely not "orders") to be hospitalized when they got cholera. Worry about fear (or fear of worry) was often at the heart of these efforts. You might make hysteria a crime, as McGrew notes of Russia, but any attempt to stop it would be to cause it. Reassurance and distraction were essential. When Berlin was threatened, the authorities made a point of keeping theaters and public amusements open, as well as schools and churches. In 1836 Bavaria went so far as to make life downright pleasant for the poor, who were to have access to unused housing.

A *feeling of freedom* was a precondition for accepting authority, yet in a climate of class antagonism, pretending all was normal when it plainly was not might backfire: distraction was deception, and might mask a deadly threat. During this age of liberal revolutions, governments were acutely aware that their power was fragile in times of cholera. Much later, in 1885, the Barcelona authorities hesitated to admit an epidemic. To announce one would cause the closing of the workplaces of 150,000, but more serious were the "republican and anarchist ideas" of these workers, "who would take advantage [of the closing] to foment a general rising for political ends."[9] It was never wholly clear that making people happy and letting them have their say and go their way lessened cholera deaths, but at least they would not go French on you. By contrast, in liberal polities like Scotland, the authorities might get away with stronger measures, like interdicting traffic into Edinburgh. In such places, investment of trust by liberal governments in their free citizens was being repaid by trust in the authority of those governments.

These changes were responses to failures of isolation-based interventions, yet to infer, as does Peter Baldwin, a learning curve overstates. The Russian response was intensely studied. Russian doctors differed on the nature of cholera, and so did the foreign colleagues studying them. That hospital staff initially seemed insusceptible to cholera suggested it was non-contagious; once a few succumbed, that was in doubt.

Medical information was not automatically medical intelligence. The visiting investigators learned what failed, but not always why. It was hard to distinguish inept administration from erroneous policy and from the variability of the disease itself. The most sober advice sent back by Western observers was that cholera could not be stopped; personal hygiene and local cleanup might minimize and mitigate, but they would not prevent.

A common recourse was to try to corral cholera with cordons, while at the same time scouring towns of refuse and of dirty animals, and feeding and clothing the poor. In the 1860s most governments would reassert control of human movement as the primary means to combat cholera. That being the case, we can as easily say that, in their under-appreciation of cholera's movement along the routes of human commerce, their predecessors in the 1840s were exhibiting a forgetting curve as much as a learning one.

Baldwin labels these pragmatic responses "Pascalian." Not knowing for sure whether cholera is contagious or non-contagious and recognizing that they cannot quickly eliminate that uncertainty, cholera authorities "play it safe," seeking to lower risks in a cost-effective way. Yet precautionary principles, risk analysis, cost–benefit thinking, and decision theory are far in the future.

This too is too rational a reading. The pragmatic empiricism versus theory and ideology dichotomy leaves out habit. Liberal or autocratic, states usually met cholera by going into their practiced epidemic response mode. Much easier to fit problem to bureaucracy than to adapt bureaucracy to problem; that would require lengthy and uncertain investigation.

Hence governments responded to the novelty of cholera by pretending it was not novel. The primary epidemic response was that for plague. Plague practice had been developed chiefly in sixteenth-century Italy. While predicated on the assumption of contagion and relying on quarantines and cordons as a first line, prevention strategies also addressed local environmental quality and individual constitution. On the approach of an epidemic, out came the scavengers' carts and the vinegar and whitewash to control smells, the sulfur and tar to alter the atmosphere. Away went the pigs and pets and as many other urban excreters as could conveniently be disposed of. Alms for the poor became a priority. As with therapeutics, the response repertoire was limited. If one method seemed ineffective, another was tried; best was to try several. This was trying known remedies, not testing, and it was much easier to add an element than to justify dropping one.

Even had there been a clear precept for determining how good was good enough, it is hard to see how they could have done better. To conceive, much less carry out, a convincing trial comparing alternative strategies required not merely statistical techniques that would not begin to exist until late in the nineteenth century, but assumptions about the constancy of disease in different times and places. Without a way to measure it, empirical success *could not matter* to governments as much as we may think it ought to have done. If, in the sixteenth century, the eclectic response to plague might represent experience leading to prudence, by the nineteenth it was expected routine: governments went through the motions, however inapplicable to the condition at hand. Many Russian cholera doctors, Baldwin notes, were "happily content with the peaceful coexistence of individual predisposition, environmental influences and [contagious] transmission."[10] The same applied to doctors elsewhere.

Cholera and community

Rulers were used to crises. In principle, they could make decisions, command minions, allocate resources. But for the first three-quarters of the nineteenth century the means at their disposal were inadequate. They might have armies and police (though in libertarian England use of either was generally unacceptable). They did not command sufficient legions of doctors or sanitary engineers, nor were there enough hospitals in the right places.

Once national borders had been breached, dealing with cholera fell to towns and villages. Indeed, to think of cholera as pandemic is misleading; rather, cholera presented as a series of local epidemics. That cholera traveled the routes of commerce was a half-truth; it rarely followed all routes. "The disease," noted the *Cholera Bulletin* of New York (1832), "has manifested a preference for one line of movement, and has rejected another, though there has been no striking difference in the amount of human intercourse between the two directions to explain the preference and rejection."[11] Some places were spared. Or they might be struck heavily or lightly.

What happened in communities mattered, often more than what states did. But communities rarely adapted easily to becoming institutions of cholera response. If states were the units of crisis, villages and towns were the units of normality, where people produced and traded, grew up and died. While states could act boldly, the problem in towns was to act at all.

Cholera forced communality on communities, argued Kingsley and Oxford's Acland. Recognition that the welfare of any was dependent on the continued health of each could bring out needed knowledge, skills, and resources. But the challenge of cholera could equally bring forth ignorance and animus, division, a false sense of invulnerability, futile gestures to stay the epidemic. As in Kingsley's Aberalva, cholera occasioned pettiness and pigheadedness. "That here government chap as the doctor sed he'd bring down to set our drains right"? "If he goes meddling with our drains, and knocking of our backyards about," say some Aberalvans, "he'll find himself over the quay…"

Usually cholera responses relied heavily on what would now be called the voluntary sector, yet in many mid-sized nineteenth-century towns local government overlapped with clubs, confraternities, or charities, or even the new local sanitary societies. Local governments were rarely prepared for the multidimensional crisis of cholera; citizens supplied both labor and resources. Examples of enthusiastic civic engagement are plentiful, from Moscow to Oxford to Palermo to St Louis.

However worthy this commitment to communality, it was insufficient, even problematic, in the eyes of some professionals. Charitable organizations to provide food or nursing might present themselves as eponymous of, and responsible to, the "public," but their "public" was often partial. As expressions of the heart, they might be wanting in competence, comprehensiveness, or continuity, and resist coordination. "We are laboring under the greatest misapprehension," wrote Albanesi of Palermo, "if we believe that committees of assistance and voluntary bands of nurses will be sufficient…"[12] Yet more specialized expertise—voluntary or professional—brought its own problems of self-legitimation, the elevation of special mission over the common good.

Then there was the problem of temporality. Communities might band together in a cholera emergency, but they would not systematically prepare for one. That was true for public authorities as well as voluntary groups. The former, complained

Albanesi, "try to do in a day" what required weeks or months. They neglected procedures, regulations, training. They then spent wastefully. Having ignored the warnings of local doctors, they were compelled to "hope for a repetition of the multiplication of loaves and fishes": it was unrealistic to think that "a badly organized and an inferior staff...badly paid" could perform "extraordinary...services which require energy, knowledge, and promptitude."[13] And, once cholera had left, its lessons were forgotten. Asked what had been done to prevent a return, a Spanish local official replied that nothing had: "This is our nature. We remember Santa Barbara only when it thunders— and it must thunder loudly—yet we curse the result. This is Spanish."[14]

As a matter of management, cholera presented four problems:

1. How should individual and community prepare?
2. How to know when cholera has truly come. People are always getting bowel diseases. Sometimes they die of them, so when do matters pass from normal to epidemic and then back to normal?
3. What to do during the epidemic. How to treat one another and outsiders; what part of normal life to hold on to and what to give up.
4. How to assess the event. And to present it to the outside world. How to measure success and failure. How to allocate blame or praise.

I take these in turn. A caveat: these are problems that arose where there *was a public* response. There was not always one. "We have here to do with Civilized Communities only," wrote Acland.[15] In some places the disease will have passed through and the deaths mounted without transgressing the normal.

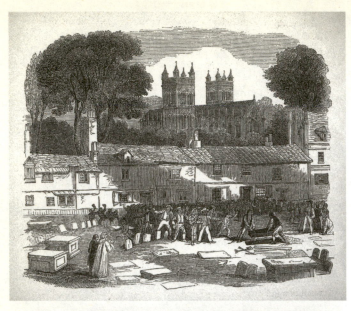

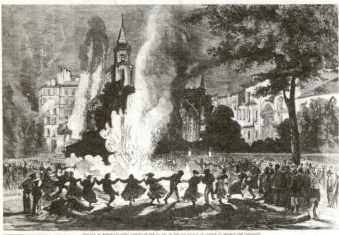

6, 7. Cholera produced many kinds of community. Above, a cholera riot, from Shapter's reflections on the 1832 cholera at Exeter. *(Wellcome Library, London)*. Below, in Marseilles in 1865, residents celebrate the purging of the epidemic air. *(Harper's Weekly, Nov. 18 1865, National Library of Medicine)*.

Preparation

What Acland called the "well-ordered habits of the Community" did not automatically operate.[16] Many did not invest their hope in community. They fled. If cholera were a matter of place and not of person, it were better not to be there. If it was contagious and one already had it, it made no difference; if not, it was best to get out of its path. In many places flight was a traditional response to epidemics; further, it meant taking control, breaking free of the cycle of hopelessness that might itself contribute to cholera.

Generally, states frowned on flight. Movement, after all, spread plague. Panicked flight of those with no place to go and nothing to fall back on might be a greater social problem, not just for the region that must temporarily absorb the fleeing, but for the place to which they returned. They might bring cholera, or another disease, back with them.

And was not flight also cowardly? Views were mixed. Kingsley saw flight as the obvious recourse for the wealthy house party set; sailing off on a yacht is prudent retreat to save valuable lives. Yet he applauds the decision to stay of the landlord, young Lord Scoutbush, as responsible aristocratism. When cholera first came ashore in Britain, in Sunderland in November 1831, Lord Londonderry stayed, conspicuously in the public eye. Civic leaders in American seaboard cities felt a similar *noblesse oblige*: one should stay even if one could flee. One Spanish medical correspondent took pride in reporting "absolutely no flight . . . complete confidence."[17]

But by the 1880s, some French, Spanish, and Italian doctors, sometimes backed by municipal authorities, were telling people to leave. They were, one suspects, recognizing abysmal cure rates. Shakespeare claimed 80,000–100,000 had left Marseilles. At Elche in Alicante, about 6,000 in a population of 14,000 fled, even though the cholera was not expected to be bad. Should we believe such numbers? Cholera deaths are hard enough to count; masses of moving persons are even harder.

Work was the chief reason to stay. Some probably left when the epidemic stopped commerce and industry, while others probably stayed because they had nowhere to go. A St Louis woman defended her decision to stay in 1850: it would be hard to get medical care in the countryside should she need it; in any case she had been assured that she could protect herself and that cholera, caught early, could be cured.

A successful defense against cholera required time and money. Aggressive preparation could be consistent with business as usual. Temporary hospitals could be identified and equipped; drugs and disinfectants stocked. A Board of Health could be established to coordinate and root out "nuisances." It might pay to watch newcomers, keeping a special eye on where they slept and what became of bedding and clothing.

The attack on nuisances required an appeal to cholera panic to destabilize sensibilitites, to make normal practices transgressive. Once common states of environment, household, or behavior could be rendered as violations of the internalized code vital to the efficient conduct of social life—made "pollutions" in Mary Douglas's terms—visceral disgust, operating through peer pressure, and, if need be, mob outrage, could be relied upon to enforce cleanliness.[18]

In many places the authorities needed no special powers to take such steps; that was what it meant to be an "authority."

Where they did, as in "house is castle" England, the laws, like the successive Nuisances Removal Acts (passed after 1847), were open-ended. The parish could act against a *"filthy* and unwholesome condition of any *dwelling-house* or other *building,"* order removal of "any *offensive* or noxious *matter, refuse, dung,* or *offal,"* or condemn "any *foul* or offensive *drain, privy,* or *cesspool.*"[19] No harm need be demonstrated; after 1855 there was to be an inspector (of nuisances) to be on active lookout for such matters. Even where principles of private property were sacrosanct, cholera could make summary inspection, designation, and seizure acceptable. Anti-cholera actions of English local authorities probably often exceeded their legal powers. Often no one complained: where communities were united, decisive action trumped quibbles about rights.

It did not follow that recognition of a need to act translated easily into unanimity of action. Sometimes there was resistance to invasive government, yet often the complaints were aimed not at public action in general but at particular acts: what was proposed was not optimal or not of highest priority. Or the costs were being unfairly distributed, or, simply, "I am not in charge." Indeed, concerns about inequitable administration were almost unavoidable. In a community where everyone's affairs were entangled with everyone else's and long had been, cholera disturbed that hoary stasis. It offered an opportunity for the cock of each dung hill to crow, perhaps for old scores to be settled. Public process—"the charming machinery of local government," in Kingsley's sarcasm—is no match, but rather a means of expressing and exacerbating conflict. In Aberalva, each attendee at a vestry meeting must speak. Whatever is said is objectionable to someone, or it sparks an irrelevant observation or devastating witticism—which may offend another. A key difficulty, Kingsley recognized, was that communal problems were expressed as accusations against individuals. These were being called upon to confess transgression of community standards, which everyone else was probably violating too.

Matters of equity were not the only impediments. Many anti-cholera actions were ambiguous in their effects on cholera. Suspension of trade would lower income, thus adversely affecting the "necessaries" of diet, clothing, and shelter, in turn undermining resistance to cholera. Urban pigs were an early target of anti-cholera campaigns. Yet, while swine might smell, they excelled as scavengers, and represented income and nutrition. In Leeds a Working Men's Pig Protection Society fought in 1853 for pig-keeping freedom. And, however dangerous "filth" might be, disturbed filth might be worse. Digging into filth released buried foulness (or germs); moving it endangered other places. The closed docks of Marseilles or Toulon were effectively sewage sumps; dredging them was exceedingly dangerous. Nuisance removal could backfire in other ways. If the scavengers' dunghills were designated nuisances, they might stop street-sweeping. Michael Sigsworth summarizes the objectionable elements: "Family life was disrupted, cleansing and nuisance removal were carried out arbitrarily, property and possessions were confiscated, damaged or stolen." Cholera would also require interruption of funeral and burial customs, a sensitive issue.[20] What is remarkable is not that there were objections, but that there were not many more.

Who was to authorize, organize, and pay for all these preparations—the relocation of middens, the fitting-out of hospitals, the stocking of calomel and quicklime? And, once cholera had come, who would direct their use, schedule and supervise hospital staff, privy inspection, and street-sweeping? Whose job was it to feed the poor, kept from their normal work? In England, cholera exposed and exacerbated incoherent administration. Among the four large towns in West Yorkshire (Hull, Leeds, Bradford, and Sheffield), Sigsworth notes, cholera authorities included municipal corporations (that is, mayor, aldermen, and council), improvement commissions, boards of poor-law guardians, parishes, highway boards, and spontaneous lay boards; rarely were there clear delineations of responsibility. Occasionally, they worked well together nonetheless.

All the more important then, the example of Acland's Oxford: for surely Oxford would respond rationally and rightly, and could indicate best practices for other places. It was neither a poor nor (then) an industrial town; its housing stock was good. Among its 27,000 was a disproportionate number of "disinterested, benevolent persons, of easy circumstances." It enjoyed "a zealous body of parochial clergy, and excellent [charitable] institutions."[21]

Under Acland's supervision, Oxford's response was indeed comprehensive. The town was systematically inspected and its nuisances removed. For medical purposes, it was divided into districts, each with an on-call doctor. They could summon nurses, while an inspector—"an old Waterloo soldier"—saw to the needs of non-stricken family members and to destruction of contaminated items (and to their valuation and replacement). The cholera doctors met nightly to reallocate labor to worst-affected districts and, noted Acland, for tea, *free* tea (small kindnesses made all the difference).

Most remarkable was Acland's "Field of Observation," a combination hospital, convalescent center, shelter for dependents of victims, and disinfection–destruction station for contaminated items. As a medical facility, the Field did not work especially well, but Acland gloried in its moral impact. Under the supervision of ladies bountiful, the dependents of victims were prayed for (at?, to?, with?) daily, and given books and needlework. The teaching was also "by the persuasion of games, and by the discipline of cleanliness." Also important was "cheerful decoration of flowers and of pictorial illustrations…to remove the horror of the pest house." Acland hoped that all these habits, prayers, hymns, games, and flowers would stick in the "widowed and fatherless homes, where they were not known before!" The insinuation is that the problematic cholera deaths are of male breadwinners, and also that their absence makes room for moral reform.[22]

More than recovery and prevention of cholera was at stake: epidemic was opportunity. Here, in the Oxford of the Oxford movement, cholera was occasion for release of pent-up charitable energy and for infliction of Christian community. Hunger, accentuated by unemployment that was due to long college vacations, was a great predisposer in Oxford, Acland insisted. Food charities quickly outstripped need. There were not merely good soup kitchens—"strong mutton broth" at the Town Hall—but "roast meat" at Christ Church. Yet relatively few showed up for it. In its anxiety to enact community, Oxford had over-reacted in areas of intimate and visible communality while neglecting the hidden problems of drainage and sewage disposal. For Acland (Kingsley too), cholera was a time to realize one's imagined community. The community—in its first form as parish—was a Christian unit. Notably, in Oxford, it was the clergy who allocated the meat. Political economy had not been forgotten: "It may be confidently stated (if any desire to know it) that extreme care was taken to control…every unnecessary expenditure."[23]

The chaos of Aberalva and West Yorkshire were probably more characteristic of English local responses to cholera than was Oxford's coordination, but, even in polities with clearer command structures, the normal units of local government were often patently inadequate. They were either too busy with other matters, lacked expertise and capacity, or failed to command respect. A common recourse was establishment of a temporary Board of Health of the local worthies: merchants, bankers, major employers. This too was a plague-response institution. Such boards usually included, but rarely were dominated by, doctors. To doctors, who often criticized them, their amateurish and even democratic ditherings were unsuited to a problem demanding a SWAT team response. Russia's error with cholera, sneered Nelson, was due to reliance on a board composed of *"merchants,* besides disinterested scientific men. A *majority* was to decide. It is easy to see that cupidity would overpower honesty; accordingly a *majority of votes* decided that purification was unnecessary."[24]

But we should be cautious. Cholera chronicles are usually the works of doctors. Roth reports that St Louis's response to the 1850 cholera was ineffective until an ad hoc emergency board was established. It had a budget of $50,000 and was made up mostly of laymen.[25] The ability of such boards to act (they did not always) came from their representativeness and ability to confront cholera in the context of all other local issues. More than the doctors, boards could appreciate that cholera was not exclusively medical. They could recognize too that the local medical profession, often an amalgam of rival systems and jealous individuals, did not always command the esteem it coveted. Nor were they disinterested: money was to be spent, much of it on them.

Contemporary chroniclers rarely discuss the finances of cholera response. Who sent the bills and who paid them? Or did physicians usually work for free during crises? The doctors on Acland's staff averaged a guinea per day, the nurses ("respectable women"), 10s. 6d. a week. But there were also inspectors, disinfectors, and registrars to be employed. In prosperous cities of reasonable size it is likely that the existing units of municipal government bore the costs. Rosenberg reports municipal expenditure on the 1832 cholera as almost $120,000 for New York, about $19,000 for Albany, and about $50,000 for Boston. These figures included fees for medical attendance. Elsewhere it was probably these boards of health, which could tap into local philanthropic networks, or even individual landlowners, who paid the costs.[26]

Arrival

"We have got the name cholera introduced into this country and we will never get rid of it."[27] One issue too important to be left to the doctors was the declaration that epidemic cholera had begun (or, equally, had ended). It was important to be prepared, and equally important not to over-react. For there were consequences. Regardless of whether cholera was deemed contagious or attributed to some environmental aberration, almost everywhere it stopped normal activity. One reads of quiet, deserted streets; illustrations, like Shapter's 1832 Exeter woodcuts (published in 1899), are strikingly bereft of people moving about. The economic losses to a stricken community were real and deep. Further, to admit the existence of cholera in a place was to create fear, which predisposed to the disease itself. Cholera denial is a common theme of cholera historians, though "cholera reluctance" would be fairer. Given the error costs, those who would proclaim an epidemic were expected to meet a high burden of proof.

In Kingsley's Aberalva, cholera comes all at once and unmistakably. But a common pattern during pandemics was of weeks or months of sporadic diarrhea preceding an outbreak: cholera's foreplay, as it were. Yet an outbreak did not always follow; whether these cases were mild cholera or something else is unclear. Thus the problem of deciding when cholera had arrived had both qualitative and quantitative elements: one had to know if it really was cholera and whether it was truly epidemic. Identification of epidemic onset was (and is) often retrospective. Once the epidemic is clearly going, it can be traced backwards. Alfred Stillé's assertion that cholera was likely to be epidemic cholera when there was a cholera epidemic going on may seem circular but it characterizes a great deal of past and present practice.[28] Needless to say, this was little help in making costly, and perhaps irreversible, decisions.

The unmistakability of cholera diagnosis has often been asserted, but these considerations suggest that it may be fruitful to revisit celebrated cases of dithering, like that of Reid Clanny, stationed at Sunderland by the British Privy Council in the spring of 1832 to watch for the coming cholera. Clanny's reputation has never recovered from his decision, made under pressure from local merchants, to diagnose the first English epidemic as common *cholera nostras*. He could not have been wrong for any right reason, it is often suggested; he must have lied, since he could not have doubted.

Certainly, cholera writers regularly asserted that they could reliably distinguish the dangerous cholera from the autumnal flux. But it is likely that we rarely hear of the clinical false positives. Unlike the skeptical Stillé, Nelson was sure he could spot the real thing. He recalled his first encounter: "while the symptoms appeared to differ only in degree [from common cholera]...there was a great difference, but what difference *words* can not point out, more than a witness can define what difference there is between two countenances." Perhaps, yet Nelson, like most other clinicians, admitted also that each of the cholera symptoms varied from mild to severe. And elsewhere he admitted that what *he* knew as common cholera did not fit the textbook description.[29] "Pro and Con; Or cholera, or No Cholera," an 1832 burlesque of doctors' disagreements, dealt with the problem:

> Violent Spasms, Rice-coloured Evacuations, and blueness of skin are unquestionable evidences of Asiatic Cholera; says Dr A.
>
> I have repeatedly seen violent Spasms, Rice-coloured Evacuations, and blueness of the Skin, in American Cholera; says Dr B.[30]

Confusion might well have been expected in the first pandemics, when epidemic cholera was new to many doctors. Yet it persisted. US consular officers were resident in foreign ports to make such determinations, yet these decisions were not being made reliably. Edward Shakespeare's great 1890 cholera report to the American government was prompted by the difficulty of detecting cholera early enough to take effective steps. In France, Spain, and Italy "prompt, vigorous, and judicious action...was paralyzed by...uncertainty concerning the real nature of the disease." In Játiva, later recognized as the focus of cholera in

Spain, "*suspicious cases*" during the winter of 1884–5 led to declarations, counter-declarations, and confusion.

> A few affirmed…that they were dealing with genuine Asiatic cholera; some insisted [it]…was nothing more than the common sporadic cholera; others declared it to be a pernicious fever of the choleraic type; many claimed that it was malignant malarial fever; yet others held that it was a kind of entero-gastritis; and not a few pretended that it was the bubonic plague, but without the boils.[31]

This was typical, Shakespeare declared. He does not rail at poor medical training in Mediterranean countries. We have no right to assume that even experienced doctors will usually have gotten it right; much reason to sympathize with Clanny, faced with a combination of high stakes and uncertain diagnosis. Governments, hearing conflicting reports from confident doctors, will have been much less sure than the confident Nelson. For Shakespeare the great promise of Koch's cholera vibrio was diagnostic. There were false alarms (or apparent false alarms), as in Hull in September 1848: cases appeared to have been imported from Hamburg, but no epidemic broke out. The eventual conclusion was that the cholera was "English." The real cholera would come the next summer.

Coping

Once cholera had clearly broken out, what to do then? Would the public cooperate? Many would not, Acland acknowledged. If even a few did not, cholera might gain entry. The responsible community did not wait for sufferers to come knocking; their diarrhea must be sought out. In mid- and late-nineteenth-century Europe, house-by-house inspections were a standard response to cholera. One thing the inspectors wanted to know was whether anyone had diarrhea, seen as an early sign of cholera. How did they find out? They asked, or, if there was anything to look at, they looked—at the condition of dwellings, and at privies or whatever form of excrement disposal/storage was being used (the water closet was a friend to privacy long before the age of marijuana). There were consequences. If they found you a little too loose, they might treat you, try to talk you into treatment, or simply take you off to a hospital. "In a quiet respectable house" Acland found soiled linen, kept under a bed for washing day by people who knew better.[32]

At the outset of the cholera era, the usual practice had been to enforce hospitalization or cleansing. By mid century this had given way to a firm but friendly approach, as it became clear that heavy-handedness led only to a detection–deception arms race. The powers of the people to mislead were great. In the early 1880s, British officials in newly occupied Egypt complained of the difficulty of getting sound sanitary information. "The Egyptians have a natural dread of being questioned" and an "unpleasant habit of stating whatever will suit themselves."[33] Yet they were hardly unique.

As it became clearer that cholera was contagious, sanitary scrutiny became ever more autocratic. Policies abandoned in the 1830s, when cholera control had been seen as repression, were being readopted in the 1880s. Added to the questioning of persons and the inspections of dwellings were the regulation of drains and diet, restraints on movement, pre-emption of public gatherings, pervasive disinfection, destruction of clothing and bedding, and curtailment of the customary rituals of death. Dr Messina outlined his response to the 1884 cholera in Vernet-les-Bains, Pyrenées Orientales:

After the appearance of the first case of cholera I urged the mayor of Vernet to have the streets cleaned, to have the heaps of manure against the sides of nearly all of the houses, and the foecal matter openly deposited in the narrow streets removed. The streets were watered every day sufficiently for the removal of all kinds of filth thrown into the public streets. I attempted, but not always with success, to cause the removal of the dejecta of cholera patients which were cast upon the manure heaps, or into the streets, or even into the gutters...by quick lime kept in the chamber pots I endeavoured to neutralize the dejecta of the cholera patients. After death I caused the cadavers to be disinfected by washing them with a strong solution of corrosive sublimate, and the clothes used by the patients to be immersed in a solution of carbolic acid. Interment was made as soon as possible, five to six hours after death. The bed furniture was burned in the open air and the houses were disinfected with sulphurous acid...I did my best to counsel the inhabitants of the infected quarter to abandon their houses and remove to a more healthy location. This measure did good through isolation of the houses and raising the morale of the unaffected and healthy population.[34]

In Vernet, population about 2000, there were only eleven cases, but ten deaths.

There were still protests, dissimulation, and other forms of resistance, but in many places, populations, now habituated to cholera's status as a public problem and sharing confidence that to act boldly was to act well, accepted and even welcomed such force. Ironically, trust in experts grew with the rise of democratic institutions. American consular officers were particularly appreciative of the absolute power of the bacteriological firemen put in charge of local epidemics by the Italian Interior Ministry. On coming to Palermo, Albanesi "immediately...assumed control of everything appertaining to the sanitary affairs of the city, and he exacted obedience to every order emanating from his office." At Genoa, Professor Mariglianao had no patience with local governments: their "carelessness" and "folly" had endangered other towns too. Imperiousness did generate resistance. In Palermo some "fled to other portions of the city... [to] escape being taken away by the authorities." Cholera spread.[35]

All that enthusiasm masked increasing recognition that cholera *must be* prevented because it *could not be* cured. Medically, the cardinal rule was to get in early and strike hard. The warrant for house-to-house inspection was to discover cases of "premonitory diarrhoea." Many physicians believed that this mild diarrhea almost always preceded cholera. Curing it would prevent its evolution into the severer form. If the members of the public could learn to surveil their bowels rigorously, to enlist professional aid at the earliest sign, cholera could be stopped. Later writers would spot the logical error. Persons with diarrheas that could be cured quickly were not in early cholera at all; they had ordinary self-limiting digestive upsets. Yet the view was plausible. If cholera were due to a transitory state of atmosphere, it followed that the peril varied in strength. One took steps to counter it as soon as one sensed its power. If it were due to a contagion, this diarrhea might signify a weakening of the bowels that would leave them unable to resist invasion. And practitioners had no way of knowing what course the disease would take. Even if cholera would not have ensued, there was no good reason to wait and see if it were going to do so.

Bold action was the only alternative to acquiescence. Physicians were in a difficult position. They had boasted—some still did—that cholera could be cured. Yet, as case-mortality rates rose, with 50 percent a mark of success, it became plain that none of the common therapies worked well. The likeliest reason for that fall is changed diagnostic categories: with "cholerine" or "choleraic diarrhea" available for milder illness, "cholera" was reserved for the more severe form. But the terms were imprecise and not uniformly adopted; the rise in mortality rates appears to have been independent of particular accounting and categorizing practices.

Cholera, like other diseases, experienced a wave of "therapeutic nihilism." By the second half of the century some physicians were advocating a wait-and-see approach to cholera, using lemonade, or even sugar water. It was not so much that these approaches worked as that more aggressive approaches worked no better. Stillé compared cholera to a severe burn: recovery was exception not rule; "officious and meddlesome treatment" was to be avoided. Nelson noted that few practitioners had "the courage to resist...[those] urging them to 'do something'." Hardly heartening! Faith in premonitory diarrhea was an alternative to such hopelessness.[36]

After

Summarizing the epidemic of 1884, the American consul in Marseilles declared that the "authorities...have done the utmost that zeal, courage, and intelligent liberality could do to stamp out the present cholera...The officers and people of this city have set a shining example of what may be done by human energy and wisdom to stay the ravages of cholera. The efforts have succeeded, under Providence, in notably diminishing the spread and fatality of the disease." A German journal asserted the "mildness" of cholera in the French Pyrenees.[37] Yet on what basis could one make such a statement?

With no way to know how bad an outbreak might have been, one could not know for sure the effects of one's intervention. When they looked back, towns could say only what they had done: how many houses inspected, nuisances removed, premonitory diarrheas cured, persons hospitalized, tons of disinfectant sloshed about. One could grouse. A Dr Chassinar complained that in the disinfection of his town, Hyères, in 1884, "the most stupid and absurd things" had been done. The authorities had defied the doctors in disinfecting willy nilly, spending so much that, when cholera returned a year later, they could afford only to wash the streets with water. "It was not noticed that the sanitary state of the population suffered," Chassinar noted.[38]

Confidence that one was acting boldly must be proof that one was acting well; there could be no other. We now know that the technical and medical solutions of nineteenth-century cholera authorities were often unwarranted. Yet there was no clear technical answer to cholera—in many ways there still is not. What was important was to have tried; that addressed the serious moral problem (of morale). Whatever the mortality, communities sought assurance that they had done what they could. At best that conviction strengthened community; perhaps it only flattered authority. Forgetting helped. Almost always, cholera epidemics were short. So too was memory.

The most common problem of representing a town's condition and achievement to the outside world was what to say about the death toll. As well as a round-numbers problem there was a real-numbers problem. We have often assumed that cholera deaths were commonly understated in order to make towns appear cleaner and healthier. Such claims are hard to check: usually the alternative figures are rumors and estimates. Sometimes cholera deaths were understated during the epidemic to avoid panic and corrected later, perhaps by interpolating excess deaths from other causes.

But there were complications. Unwillingness to admit cholera might mean missed cases in the weeks preceding the epidemic, while during it there might be a corresponding tendency to diagnose other conditions as cholera. Noting that bowel diseases occurred inversely to cholera in Calcutta, Shakespeare posited that "cholera is frequently registered as bowel complaints." He did not mention that the reverse was probably true as well, as in Trieste in 1886, where "during the past three months no cases of Diarrhea...have been reported, all such illness being classified as cholera."[39]

One must also factor in the tendency of rumor to grow. Cholera brought about boasting; there was competition for commemoration—"you think you suffered, we..." Of the St Louis epidemic of 1849, a correspondent asserted that "no other city either in this country or Europe has at any time suffered so much from cholera." With the passage of time, notes Roth, cholera's "virulence seemed to grow in the minds and imaginations of those who had witnessed it." Hence cholera denial might be followed by cholera kitsch. Writers could help readers imagine the cholera sublime. To have passed through the epidemic made one a hero; and the measure of heroism was the rarity of survival.[40]

Remarkably, while there might be scientific interest in finding first cases, recrimination was rarely a conspicuous part of a community's post-cholera priorities. Those who had denied cholera did not apologize; generally it was assumed that the authorities had done what they could. More important was the rebuilding of lives. In many places ordinary life was hard enough even without cholera. A physician in a Spanish village wrote to Shakespeare: "In this country we live from hand to mouth, and do not at all remember past fears or take account of the future."[41]

Why can't the English teach their subjects how to …

By the mid 1880s cholera recrimination (in the name of prevention) was an international issue, however. Between 1883 and 1887 a pandemic circled the globe. Cholera came (probably for the first time) to the southern cone of South America; it reached New Zealand and Australia. Largely bypassing Britain, the USA, and Germany, the early stages of this fifth pandemic have been overlooked in cholera's social history. It was important in its scientific history: in 1883–4, in Egypt and in India, Koch's team isolated the cholera microbe.

Steam and Suez made cholera an international issue. Beginning in 1851, a series of international sanitary conferences sought consensus on cholera control. Occurring every few years, these conferences were no regular series. Each resulted from a nation's decision that a forum was needed to address some aspect of cholera management (while designated "sanitary," they focused almost entirely on cholera). Each worked out its own protocol for debate and decision. Before 1892, their resolutions had no binding force; even after they were not enforceable. Most important were quarantine and inspection issues. Almost always it was the British who resisted. Whatever was decided, Britain did what it wanted.

As at the community level, cholera was not inherently a medical or a scientific problem. Cholera policy was about trade, and behind that about colonies, alliances, and power. Cholera science had an ambiguous status in the deliberations; it was hardly irrelevant but decidedly secondary. Nations sent medical representatives to the conferences (though not necessarily their greatest experts), but increasingly they were there to work out "technical" issues. In the 1885 Rome Conference scientists did not speak at plenary sessions, much less vote. Cholera was too important to be left to the doctors, who differed on central issues and represented the tentativeness of science.

While British diplomats exercised their tergiversative talents, by the mid 1880s most governments and most experts operated as if cholera were transmissible. Pandemics were more than dots on a map. It had long been plain that epidemic cholera followed paths of human movement; most now presumed that an infective agent moved in infected humans and in their personal articles, such as clothing and bedding. In the USA in 1873 and in Europe in 1884, small pieces of packed-away clothing were safely transported across oceans only to explode into continent-wide epidemics.

The range of response to contemporary cholera science can be gauged by comparing ultra-contagionist South America with sanitarian Britain. Cholera came late to southern South America. Jungles, mountains, and deserts impeded its spread; trade was funneled through a few great ports whose health officers took their work seriously, and the great capitals of Buenos Ayres and Montevideo were well kept. The handling by the Uruguayan authorities of the Italian ship *Matteo Bruzzo* indicated what could and should be done. During its voyage from Genoa, obscure diseases broke out, and were diagnosed as colic, cramps, anemia, and finally cholera. That recognition led to the ship being sent back to Italy without being allowed to unload in any South American port. In Robert Koch's view (and that of the Uruguayan medical press), it had no business even trying to land passengers; its captain, like so many, was trying to deceive. The *Matteo Bruzzo* case was not unique; during the next decades several Italian ships would be turned back, with a total of 522 onboard cholera deaths. When cholera came to Argentina, it was from a single lapse in similarly admirable vigilance, the expedited unloading of the *Perseo*, also from Italy, because it carried a senior Argentinian official.

From Argentina, cholera crossed to Chile. It bypassed guards on the Andean passes—jumped over or floated past a triple cordon surrounding the remote Chilean valley in which it first broke out. Peru closed its ports to ships from Chile, cutting off all eastern Pacific trade. On the Atlantic side, Brazil and Uruguay instituted quarantine "against" Argentina. Here too trade stopped.

All this for an epidemic that was apparently mild, at least in the well-kept capitals where American consular officers dictated their reports. The Buenos Aires officer disparaged the "grossly exaggerated reports" about his city that were coming from Montevideo. "A mild sporadic" cholera, largely confined to inmates of an asylum, was in the city, but there had been more deaths from the supposedly tame *cholera morbus* in each of the preceding twelve years. Yet other American diplomats in Argentina were repeating rumors of devastation in the interior: Mendoza—"almost decimated"; 500 cases a day in Tecuman. But, as the Montevideo consul admitted, "information" was really rumor: even in the city of one's residence, one could not be sure what was going on.

Argentina and Uruguay had put lives above trade. Had it worked? Shakespeare judged that their governments should have acted more quickly. Yet the very documents he published showed how hard it had been to figure out what was happening until it had happened. There were cases of over-reaction. In 1886 cholera broke out on the *Plata*, while it awaited permission to unload. The Buenos Aires port authorities thought there might be yellow fever aboard, even though it had halted offshore at the suspect ports only to offload cargo. The cholera came while the ship was in port. Passengers, exhausted by sea-sickness, filth, bad food, and worry over whether they would be allowed to land, had hauled up contaminated water from the foul estuary.

International control of cholera was only as strong as the weakest link. Usually that was Britain. Even though the cholera had come on an Italian ship, *El Monitor Medico* blamed Argentina's cholera on Britain: "the English introduced cholera into Europe, and Buenos Aires received the disease."[42] Excoriations of British practices abound in the literature of the 1880s and 1890s. A French delegate at the 1894 Sanitary Conference called British India "the factory of cholera." Even if Britain were not guilty of willful murder, as masters of the seas, the British were uniquely able to remedy the problem. Yet the captains singled out for overlooking cholera were usually British. Beyond complaints of laxity are implicit accusations of genocidal neglect: in pursuit of greed, the British care nothing for lives.[43]

Surely *we* are not to blame for *your* cholera, British authorities replied. Cholera was the product of many factors: even if a mobile infectious something sometimes comes from India (not an admission, mind you), there would be no cholera without filth and poverty. Even if valid, Koch's discovery was irrelevant. Tendentious? Probably so. As an island nation, Britain could readily secure its ports, and in fact did so through a system of port sanitary administration and surveillance of arrivals during their first days ashore. Why could they not accept others' needs for similar safeguards? Shakespeare found the British stance hypocritical and cowardly; Stillé thought it dishonest and immoral: if "all nations had honestly carried out the rules pre-scribed by experience for the exclusion of disease...there can be little doubt that its ravages would ere this *have been confined to that region in which it originated.*" (Stillé would save the world by sacrificing India.) British cholera deception ranked high in the annals of infamy: "the ethics which justified the introduction of opium into China by the English and the American gift of alco-hol to the Indian...[were] only paralleled by...official protests against cholera quarantines."[44]

In broadest terms, the British answer was that prudence, practicality, and flexibility did not constitute hypocrisy. No nation should trust external defenses alone; to emphasize inter-nal improvements—that is, sanitation that would stanch any incipient cholera—was simple common sense. Moreover, it was foolish to found public-health policy on any assumption of universal human virtue. One dealt with people as they really were, not as we would want them. Cordons and quarantines, John Simon had observed, *would* be evaded. Travel and trade *would* occur; constraint simply invited violation. A wholly reac-tive cholera policy was invariably too late and too weak, and only as strong as its most inept or corrupt functionary. Despite all the anger at British imperiousness, many acknowledged that Simon was right. They also respected Britain's achievement in cholera control. Sanitized Britain, they were often reminded, had had no cholera since 1866.

But how serious was partial failure? Stillé held that even par-tial border controls were preferable to "fatalism" or to capitu-lation to the "Mammon-worshippers."[45] Yet, when it came to germs, the partial-protection argument fell to pieces, insisted Albanesi. Cholera came in tiny units—"30,000,000,000 of these creatures hardly weigh a milligram when dry"—and they could multiply. Hence the common analogy with customs inspection could not hold. One need only consider the "destruction which the thousandth part of a milligram of microscopic beings can cause," realize that they could survive for long periods, and cross human barriers on "a garment...a rag, or in a little water" to appreciate the dilemma. Since with respect to microbes the issue was multiplicability not mass, quarantines were futile.[46]

If quarantines and cordons were sometimes adopted, it was not because lives were valued over lucre, but because they were cheaper than the British alternative of comprehensive sanitation. Cholera crises provided a brief window to push sanitary measures many thought desirable. Usually it was too brief. In Messina in 1886, the Interior Ministry's cholera czar, Professor Canalis, created a system of "well" ships to bring safe water from the mainland. So patently absurd a stopgap was intended to spur the building of pipes to convey spring water from the mountains into the city. In Naples and Palermo cholera prompted the razing of bad housing and the widening of streets. And yet in Albanesi's view what Italy really needed was what England had, something akin to the Public Health Act of 1875, which set out expectations and provided mechanisms through which every town could (and must) work steadily to secure its own sanitary salvation.

That did not happen. Cholera and other epidemics returned regularly. Misery persisted. Effective action was so hard precisely because the problem was so extensive and pervasive. How to end cholera in Toulon? It could not really be done, reflected the American consul: "The sanitary defects...are so radical and so numerous...parts of the town would need to be entirely demolished and rebuilt."[47] We should reflect that the British sanitary infrastructure being touted as the model to which every town should aspire was in fact the product of rare economic conditions that cannot be readily replicated. Using the vehicle of long-term loans, Victorian towns spent hugely on public works. Tax rates rose, but prosperity grew faster. There would be similar spates of municipal improvement elsewhere, but not everywhere. It could not be assumed that sanitation would somehow pay for itself. Britain had spent $300 million on sanitation in a single decade, Shakespeare noted, yet still relied on border controls. "Assuredly the United States of America, where, as a rule, the hygienic laws and organizations are very crude and insufficient, could ill afford…to trust her safely to such idealistic means of protection."[48]

Could the world ever be both busy and cholera free? A cordon-based response seemed the only option for many nations. Reactive responses were costly, but systematic transformation was costlier. And even the British seemed unable to sanitize India. They protested that they were trying; Indian cholera was indeed shifting from city to countryside during the early twentieth century. But progress was slow, and incidence and mortality both remained high.

What resulted was a "band-aid" program of control, pragmatic but strategic. The elements were hardly new—border controls; inspections at ports of landing (and of embarkation, an American innovation in 1881) for ships and trains; the requirement that the masters of ships log illnesses and causes of deaths (cholera had its own flag, distinct from other quarantine flags). In what Crosby has called the "neo-Europes"—the Americas, South Africa, and the Antipodes—cholera would be controlled by rising levels of sanitation, domestic hygiene, general medical oversight of populations, and targeted border controls, concentrating on poor immigrants, especially during epidemics. Mostly, these would keep epidemics from getting started, while allowing great freedom of travel and trade. Elsewhere, i.e. Asia the controls would be much more rigorous. Quarantines (though usually five rather than forty days) might be necessary. But this was permissible; life in Asia was slower. Holding back Asian travelers until they were reliably cholera free was no great burden. One liberated some by controlling others.

East is east and west is west

The enormous concern for international regulation did not occur in a vacuum; it arose in response to a particular geopolitical problems. For, after 1867, the twain did meet regularly, at one spot: along the Red Sea and the Suez Canal. There at a different time each year (owing to the lunar calendar) Muslim pilgrims converged on their way to the holy sites around Mecca and later diverged on their way home. In doing so, they crossed or paralleled the main commercial and colonial route between Europe and Asia. Accordingly, for roughly a half century, the Hajj was seen by Europeans primarily as an occasion for the collection, amplification, and dissemination of cholera; to a remarkable degree, the disease was associated with Islam, though Britain was seen as enabler.

There had been cholera in Mecca before the opening of the Suez Canal, but it had never occasioned much comment. The first major Hajj-related epidemic was that of 1865–6, as the Canal was being dug. The cholera was said to have stricken about 10,000 of the 90,000 pilgrims. Thereafter Hajj-based epidemics were noted on a regular basis—eight more had occurred by 1895, including annual outbreaks in 1889–91. In 1893 it was estimated that 15 per cent of the pilgrims had died from cholera.

Cholera among Hindu pilgrims could be seen as Britain's problem, but Muslim pilgrimage was an international issue. Islam was a world religion; returning pilgrims might spread cholera almost anywhere. The holy sites themselves were mainly in Ottoman territory, but the European powers expected little from the "sick man of Europe." Moreover, the Hajj was off limits to infidels, and, for most of the century, that meant to European cholera investigators. Before 1895, by which time there was a health officer in Mecca and some measure of acceptable sanitary accountability, the Hajj had been a subject of sanitary sensationalism, much of it based on the explorer Richard Burton's 1853 exposé. There were reasons for concern. Many pilgrims arrived in Arabia exhausted, underfed, and at the mercy of guides and other purveyors. Mecca and Medina had insufficient housing, water, or sanitation for so many; it was difficult to carry out the hygienic practices of Islam in a satisfactorily hygienic fashion. The emergence of steam navigation and later railroad service both allowed more penitents to undertake the journey and accelerated the transmission of cholera.

Prevented from intervening directly in Arabia, European authorities tried to affect the rates and routes of traffic in and out of the holy region. On the west, Mecca was close to the Red Sea port of Jedda, and thence to Africa, the Levant, and Europe. Some suggested that steam navigation made access too easy and that steps should be taken to stop the poor or ill from setting out.

Before steam, pilgrims from the east and north had come overland in caravans. At the 1866 Conference the French proposed a return to that practice: to block return by sea of pilgrims during cholera epidemics and instead to force all to experience the lazaretto of desert travel. The cholera—and those who carried it—would not survive. But, if the pilgrims must suffer, again it was the British who were to blame. Like all cholera, Mecca's came from India; the British controlled most shipping in the Indian ocean (and even more in the Persian Gulf). They occupied Egypt and managed the canal that could bring cholera so quickly to Europe. The Persian delegate protested, not because that would bring cholera across Persia, but at the audacity of subjecting (Muslim) religious practice to infidel public health (and commercial) concerns. Opposed by Britain, Russia, Persia, and Turkey, the proposal passed. It was unenforceable and ignored.

The chief practical strategy of the 1880s was to seal off commercial and military traffic from the pollution of the pilgrims. Westbound ships could have no contact with land during their passage through the Red Sea and the Canal. At the same time, both arriving and returning pilgrims were to be quarantined. One station was at Kamaran Island, where you had to pay 10 piasteres for your inspection (under dreadful conditions); another, for surveillance of returning African pilgrims, was at the Suez port of Tor, and it was backed up by a cordon across north-eastern Egypt. By these means commerce could be protected from the frivolous practice of religion: "however worthy," pilgrimages, noted an Italian delegate to a Sanitary Convention, were not an "indispensable social necessity like commerce." As the Persian delegate pointed out, the whole approach—the attempt to police the long fuzzy borders of interior Asia, to control its mobile and cosmopolitan populations—was unrealistic. If Europe wanted to protect itself, it was in a much better position to apply quarantines to its own discrete and defensible borders.[49]

The British, meanwhile, were denying that cholera really did come from India. How could we be so sure? Cholera had never reached Europe from Mecca or by ship from Mumbai or Bengal, they claimed. If it moved, it came overland. Three explanations were offered for the cholera that broke out in Darmietta in the Nile delta in 1883: first, that it came from Egyptian colliers working on vessels that traded with Mumbai, second that it was a holdover from a modest 1882 outbreak introduced by pilgrims returning from Mecca, and, third, that it was generated from indigenous Egyptian filth. Darmietta's governor took the first view. He would, noted an English investigator, W. I. Simpson; he hated the English and loved filth. French and German investigators (including Koch's team) sided with him.

They reached these conclusions without evidence, Simpson protested. Those accused of introducing cholera could not have done: they were not in the right places at the right times, and/ or they did not have the disease. Their guilt was simply association with Mumbai. None of that mattered, insisted Shakespeare: Indian importation might not have been "absolutely proven," yet "there can be no reasonable doubt"; there was "no other rational explanation." Plausible deniability, after all, was the watchword of British cholera policy.[50]

Yet, thanks to Koch, it would be possible within a few years to explain such anomalies and provide the proof that Shakespeare had not been able to offer. The immediate significance of Koch's discovery of the comma bacillus was neither therapeutic nor prophylactic, but diplomatic. Culturing marked the coming of proof to the domain of lies. Without an unimpeachable authority to detect cholera, the world had lived in constant fear of any body, any cargo. Henceforth health and trade could be reconciled. As Shakespeare explained, "if...the diagnostic significance of the 'comma-bacillus' be established, its practical value must be well-nigh incalculable"; if not, *we do not at present know*

144

how to recognize a genuine epidemic cholera in time to safely guard the people against its deadly power." Lives were secondary, "insignificant when compared with the loss of incalculable millions of treasure from the paralysis of industry and commerce."[51]

A surprising finding of cholera culturing was the asymptomatic carrier. "Comma bacillus" did not always equate to cholera symptoms; the bug could be riding harmlessly in anyone's guts. If at first this was cause to doubt Koch's conclusions, it soon became a basis for redefining cholera and health status in microbiological rather than clinical terms. But culturing techniques could make the guts talk, however innocent their owner might appear to be. If the apparently healthy could infect others, there was reason to culture not only those who had been in contact with cholera victims, but those who had been in contact with the asymptomatic carriers. Indeed, with a sufficient cadre of bacteriologists, every traveler's excreta *might be* cultured, and the microbial fifth columnists rooted out and destroyed.

Plainly, the evolution of bacteriological technique into the common currency of contagiousness had transformed cholera citizenship. The imagined community of Kingsley and Acland became moot—heroic citizenship was no substitute for a suitable laboratory and capable technicians. Towns themselves were irrelevant except when cholera-bearers escaped from them. Instead, the new units were persons and nations, with the former seen as an unfortunate interference in the smooth operation of the latter. If courage were no longer relevant, veridicality and commitment to the common good (represented as willingness to squat and provide a sample) were.

For now one's bowels were not merely one's neighbors' business, they were the world's affair. Observing disembarking Muslim pilgrims at the Tor quarantine station in November

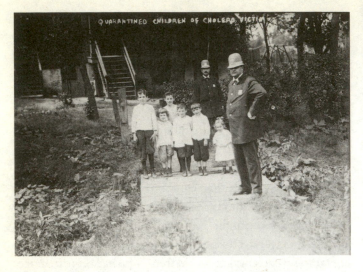

8. Cholera quarantines were serious business, even for those who were merely associated with sufferers. (*GG Bain collection, Library of Congress*)

1883, the great Koch saw several who were "strikingly weak and ill...scarcely...on shore before many sought the latrines, and *a glance at their evacuations showed at once* that they were suffering"— not in fact from cholera, but from dysentery. There was cholera, however, although the ship's surgeon had admitted only a few deaths from "senile debility."[52] Here was the medical "gaze" so beloved by Michel Foucault quite literally being magnified.

Indeed, the problem of how to implement the enormous diagnostic power of Koch's bacteriology was profound. Initially, the obvious use seemed to be to culture the uncultured, isolate the infected, and hold them until clean. But, beyond singling out persons who had been in places where cholera was rife, who should be subjected to the lengthy and degrading inspection, made to hang around at a border long enough till some busybody bureaucrat had decided one's bowels were well and truly pure? Generally carriers had to postpone their journeys until they had passed three clean stools, and even this might not prove their innocence. Around 1910 there were large-scale cholera screenings: in Egypt (of course), but also along the German–Russian border, at the ports of Amsterdam and Rotterdam, and at Naples among emigrants to the United States. Few carriers were found: 3 in 5,200 on the German–Russian border, 7 of 7,338 on ships arriving at Amsterdam and Rotterdam from the Baltic, 12 of 2,000 at Naples. In active cholera zones, among those in contact with cholera sufferers, positive results were much higher (for example, 50 per cent in Austria).

Here, at long last, was the possibility for evidence-based public-health administration. But the examinations were expensive, time-consuming, and unpleasant. It was not clear that positive results meant much or that negative results could be trusted. If the comma bacillus did not show up on ordinary stool culture, it might still be hiding in other organs and would reappear upon administration of a purgative. Evasion was possible: those with dirty guts could buy or borrow the feces of those with clean guts. Systematic culturing of travelers' excreta did not become routine, except for certain populations. Those who counted would not put up with it, even if that meant the continuation of cholera. The international sanitary bodies were unenthusiastic. They left states to make their own policies, but the general view, reiterated in 1926, was that the cost of surveillance was "absolutely out of proportion to the danger incurred."[53]

In principle, because it could separate the safe from the dangerous, bacteriology could liberalize. In practice, it did not. The bogey of the asymptomatic carrier served to reinforce the standard view—all from Bengal—rather than to challenge it. No matter if there seemed no evidence of contacts; cholera might still be hitchhiking from bowel to mouth to bowel, crossing the world (from India) with no one noticing. It appeared that the vibrio could survive in the gut for at least eight months. Since all this was known already, there was really no need to test. In this scientistic racisim, Indian origins would be reason enough for suspicion.

What was done on behalf of bacteriology fell far short of what might have been. However costly and inconvenient universal screening, there had been reason to think (at least given the knowledge of the time) that it might be the means to eradicate the disease. There is an irony here. For most of a century the vigorous response to cholera had exceeded what science could warrant. That response to cholera had been part of a wave of moral, social, and sanitary reform, part of a great clamor for human freedom. Action had gone far beyond knowledge. Now there was knowledge, but the indicated action exceeded political possibility. You could stop cholera, but people would not like it, and it would not pay, and it would inconvenience trade. That century of struggle had only revealed the indomitable rule of capital.

Cholera declined, following the coming of bacteriology, though not quickly. Each of the nineteenth-century responses to cholera—chaos-induced conscience, community, and culture plates—probably contributed to its retreat everywhere but in South Asia. Remarkably, after all the attempts to coerce, condescend to, and cajole them, citizens did come to enjoy to some degree the rewards of a moralized bacteriology in which it is recognized that anyone may be carrying cholera germs and that there is an obligation to protect others from those germs. Germs are to be the great leveler. Still, that inclusion—of places

where deadly infectious disease usually existed only in principle—would come at the expense of the radical exclusion—of
places and peoples where cholera was (or was perceived to be)
still common. South Asia would continue to suffer a cholera
stigma; it would later spread to Africa and Latin America. But
elsewhere cholera would be a matter for history and for science.
Nice and tidy, in both cases.

IV

~~~

CHOLERA CONFUSES

To historians, and equally to researchers, the "science"—the very word is contested—of cholera before the great age of bacteriology has seemed a vast wasteland. Why did authors waste their time on tons of treatises that, but for a short work by John Snow, represent a nil knowledge gain? Had pandemic cholera arisen in 1917 rather than 1817, would we have had to repeat that century of groping?

Calling this earlier period pre-scientific (or pre-paradigmatic) is not such a bad idea—at least if we can avoid the usual concomitants: that, in the face of a rapid, deadly, and terrifying entity, the unhurried rigor of science is obviously the best response. Cholera has given us exemplars of scientific method—Snow and Koch—but the philosophy of cholera is not of science alone, but rather of the entanglement of the epistemic and the ethical. Our tendency to read cholera's history as progressive, if ever so slowly before 1884, reflects a familiar faith in applied science: basic biological knowledge alone will allow an adequate response; before bacteriology there was none. And yet, to imagine a public waiting patiently for a biomedical science that can barely be imagined will not do.

More than just a problem of science, cholera was a threat to order. In an emergency, bold action mattered more than criticism and caution. Like the other arts of medicine, responding to epidemics was a matter of judicious deployment of traditional modalities. Research was chancy. Even if one were lucky enough to hit on the key variables of cholera incidence, the demand for data might be insatiable and the problem of adequate analysis insurmountable. What may seem oversimplification worked well enough; it had to; there was no alternative.

Of course the cholera authorities did talk the talk of "science," the "moral and legal trump card," as Frank Snowden puts it.[1] Science beat rights, customs, contracts, and ideologies, and was the best means of confidence creation. Familiar tropes abound: elevation of one's own experience over others' verbosity; enlistment of qualified witnesses; insistence that one's truths arise from the fullness of facts or the exhaustion of possibility; that one's methods are uniquely authoritative. The tone may be sober, but rigor is rare, as is any sense of partiality or tentativeness. Instead, iconoclasm reigns: almost everything important about cholera is known, and by us, say authors: we are in position to act.

The concern here is to make sense of, even to defend, the rejected and reviled pre-bacteriologial cholera inquiry. I represent it in terms of two dimensions: the multiplicity of legitimate questions and the imperative for authority. It helps to split the discussion into two periods—before and after 1860. At that time there are new theories, and fresh insights about cholera, notably John Snow's, and a new approach in India. The watershed of 1884—Koch—opens the next chapter.

Paradigms and positions

Questions of cholera's essential nature and causation/transmission dominate nineteenth-century discussions. Only therapeutics rivaled. The contest between "contagionists" (proto-germ theorists and eventual winners) and anticontagionists ("miasmatists," "localists," or sanitarians, who blamed cholera on bad smells or mysterious vicissitudes of climate or geology), is usually presented as enduring and unproductive. The dichotomy is ultimately unhelpful: it assumes that there is only one question to be answered and only one dimension of distinction.

Often, what appear to be antithetical positions are answers to different questions. Five are variously begged, confused, conflated, or subsumed one within another:

1. Is this "cholera" always potentially within the body or must it come from without? Is it a disease entity or simply a common physiological aberration? If it is a disease entity, how does the disease work?

2. How, when, and why did the pandemic disease ultimately begin?

3. How does it come to affect particular places? How is it transmitted?

4. Why, in those places, does it affect some and not others?

5. What accounts for its periodicity? Why does it go, and where does it go?

Along with asking different questions and theorizing different answers, authorities disagreed about the standards of good science. Some were happy theorizing about entities (like "germs") that were not directly accessible. Others ("positivists") preferred sticking to the observable. They sought correlations; were reluctant to speculate about mechanisms. Some highlighted "remote causes"—temporal, spatial, and social factors—while others studied more "proximate" causes, the mechanisms that manifested the illness.

Modern cholera science incorporates all these questions and approaches as the agendas of distinct collaborative disciplines. Nineteenth-century cholera authors were usually privileging some, often arbitrarily, and ignoring, ridiculing, or talking past those who were privileging others.

Table 4.1 summarizes pre-1860 views in terms of three positions (less coherent schools of theory and practice than heuristics): postivist anticontagionism, miasmatist anticontagionism, and contagionism. After 1860 there would be greater convergence, with most accepting some form of "contingent" contagionism. An exception would be a distinct brand of an Anglo-Indian positivism that persisted into the early twentieth century.

Table 4.1. Positions and questions on cholera, 1820–1860

Questions	Positivist anticontagionism	Miasmatist anticontagionism	Contagionism
1. Is this cholera always potentially in the body or must it come from without?	It is nothing other than its symptoms which, as *cholera nostras*, come often from a combination of climate, diet, and fatigue.	It must come from without.	It must come from without.

(Continued)

Table 4.1. Continued

Questions	Positivist anticontagionism	Miasmatist anticontagionism	Contagionism
2 How, when, and why did the disease ultimately begin?	"It" did not begin because "it" does not exist—the impression of an epidemic is a statistical artifact.	It has come about from some complex chemical condition of earth or atmosphere, ultimately global, but in some respects local too.	It has always existed perhaps, but we do not have to answer this.
3. How does it come to affect particular places?	Since there is no "it," apparent movement is not interesting: there are collective experiences of climate, diet, and fatigue: these may move.	Its movement may reflect changing states of atmosphere or soil; it may move with human victims who poison their local environments.	It moves in, and with, human carriers.
4. Why, in those places, does it affect some and not others?	Since there is no "it," there is nothing to explain. Variance is the primary datum. Of course people vary.	The environment and the human constitutions that manifest it vary constantly. People vary in degrees of predisposition.	Some are not exposed or not exposed sufficiently heavily; others may be unsusceptible. And the background of environmental conditions may be more or less dangerous.

5. Why does it go away, and where does it go to?	Since there is no "it," "it" cannot go anywhere: cholera symptoms persist in greater or lesser degrees always.	The environment changes; we lower our degree of predisposition by changing it and ourselves.	It runs out of susceptible victims; but we do not really know.

To each camp, these answers implied a distinct response strategy. But there were some overlaps. Contagionists sought in the first place to control movement and isolate the ill, but also to reinforce mental and physical state and disinfect person and surroundings. Miasmatic anticontagionists sought to control the environment; also to reinforce mental and physical state (possibly by isolating the ill), and to disinfect. Positivists emphasized mental and physical state, which might reflect environmental condition, and in turn to invite disinfection, or some more fundamental social change.

Positivist anticontagionism

As noted earlier, before the nineteenth century "cholera" was primarily a clinical concept—a flux that was seasonal or due to indiscipline of diet. There was no expectation of a common cause; the term simply collected similar clinical phenomena. That view rejected contagion, but it rejected any other form of specific cause too, including "miasms," a term that often covered all manner of atmospheric factors postulated to cause cholera. Even when the new epidemic form arrived, cholera did not quickly become a specific disease entity with a discrete cause. The older clinical *cholera morbus* meshed remarkably well with the positivism of the most progressive medical thinkers of the day, the Paris clinicians. Children (or adults) of the revolution, they would strip medicine of obscurantist theory and stick to clinical, epidemiological, and pathological fact. The people's pathology would forsake the imagined humors for demonstrable lesions in the tissues (the new units of anatomy) that one saw on post-mortem dissection, but it would still accommodate multiple causes.

For them, cholera was in the first place a life-threatening gastroenteritis. It was always potentially present (Q1). Normally the guts were in stasis; fluids came and went, but blood volume and composition were stable, and the bowels were neither loose nor compacted. In cholera all this went awry. To say that cholera resembled poisoning was a statement of analogy only, not of cause. The analogy was important. With poisons, one could isolate, measure, experiment. Cholera was intoxication, but not necessarily by a single poison or episode of poisoning.

Following the lead of Newton, the rigorous reasoner would attribute each cholera to the sum of destabilizing influences on the gut. Other questions, posited on the gratuitous assumption of an underlying essence, were question-begging. Even if cholera's epidemic profile, its waxing and waning and tracing of lines of human movement, suggested something non-random at work, still there was no need to hypothesize a single necessary specific cause, though, as we shall see, positivist epidemiology could warrant the inference of contagion.

There was positivist epidemiology as well as positivist pathology. Its touchstone was the "epidemic constitution," articulated by the seventeenth-century English physician Thomas Sydenham, following Hippocratic precedents. The determinants of epidemics were many. Some were unknown, possibly unknowable. They might include astral, atmospheric,

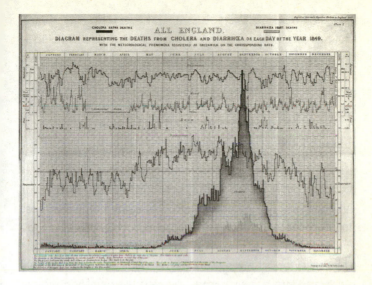

9. Cholera was a forcing ground for new modes of data presentation, as in this chart correlating cholera and diarrhea deaths with meteorological variables. It was hoped that novel presentations might suggest inferences that would not have been apparent otherwise. (*Wellcome Library, London*)

or geophysical factors as well as human activities. Hence periodicity (Q5) was a matter of a rare conjunction of conditions, which together constituted the "constitution." The term was a placeholder—less answer than advertisement of how little was known. To think of an "epidemic constitution" as an obscure something flying around with a tag of "cholera poison" misses the sense. It links the concept to the wrong question.

Paris was the capital of scientific medicine, but many of the foreign students who came to study there took home the spirit of rigor. In England, William Farr's Paris training would be reflected in his efforts to infer statistical laws of cholera incidence. Farr was no purist; from his statistics, he would also infer the operation of a cholera miasm, and later a cholera "zyme," which in turn looks to us like a cholera germ. Rarely were positivists dead set against theories. But they were in no hurry; speculation was the poison of all reasoning.

Miasmatic anticontagionism

The miasm concept that Farr and many others were applying to cholera in the 1830s and 1840s was founded in an analogy to malaria. Its fevers, recurring in three- or four-day cycles, and its occurrence in epidemics suggested some manner of specific cause, perhaps a special quality of, or entity within air, a "miasm." As malaria was linked to swamps, "miasm" became a placeholder for whatever it was that rose from festering marshes and seeped into cottages. From plague times onward, the term had been stretched to refer to emanations from rotting urban filth, including human excrement, which might cause other diseases. Cholera might arise from a specific aerial entity.

Yet the term remained vague. Along with Farr, most of the prominent English sanitarians, such as Edwin Chadwick, Thomas Southwood Smith, and John Sutherland, deployed the term. "Miasm" was weighted more toward specificity than "epidemic constitution." Yet, with its referent unknown, "miasm," like "cholera" itself, might simply be a word. "Malaria" itself might simply be a generic physiological aberration, known as fever, which at other times was expressed as typhus or cholera.

Do we know what a writer meant by "miasm"? Sometimes. In the later 1830s Southwood Smith was emphasizing a generic (and positivist) "miasm," and seeing cholera as a kind of fever. A decade or two later, he, like Farr and most others, was using the term for something akin to a specific airborne entity that caused a specific disease. It was beginning to seem likely that there were different miasmata. That from decaying plants produced malaria; that from decaying animal matter produced cholera. In such a view, cholera did represent a distinct invasion. Its emergence, rise, and fall could be attributed to the concentration or rarefaction of the cholera miasm. Yet it is not always clear that users of the term are sure what they mean or feel a need to choose among what seem to us exclusive alternatives. We, who happily use "electron" and other terms of ambivalent referent, have no right to grouse.

The process by which miasm generated disease was "infection." To us, "contagion" and "infection" refer to the same class of diseases. But in the early nineteenth century they were often antitheses. At its core, contagion implied touch; infection, transmission through (and as) tainted air. But the gap would narrow. Did not breath or emanations touch? If "miasm" owed its special malign power to someone who had suffered from cholera, whose essential qualities lived on in the decaying bodily products of the victim, miasmatic anticontagionism became a form of "contingent contagionism," a loose concept that would come to dominate in the second half of the century.

Contagionism

Today most read "contagion" as "living germ." Yet none of the three distinct models/contexts of contagion in play before 1860 was the direct ancestor of the scientific bacteriology of Pasteur and Koch.

First was the ancient hypothesis of *contagium animatium*—ludicrous adhocery to many of the best early nineteenth-century biomedical scientists. It was true that microscopic parasites for a few diseases had been identified, particularly worms. But as a hypothesis about disease in general (or even a class of diseases), it bordered on tautology: disease existed when its (invisible, inaccessible) cause existed. Prior to development of techniques for discriminating, isolating, maintaining, and experimenting with microscopic life, consideration of their roles was as facile and as sterile as speculation on the doings of hypothetical extraterrestrial beings.

One could, of course, compare drawings, hoping to correlate forms with diseases. When, in 1849, the Bristol microscopists Frederick Brittan and J. G. Swayne claimed, in conjunction with the epidemiologist William Budd, that they had found a fungus that caused cholera, the claim was quickly refuted by other microscopists who asserted that the organism was not exclusive to cholera. Even had it been, there was no obvious reason to assume that it was cause, not consequence.

Uneasiness with the facility with which anyone with a microscope might "discover" the agent of a disease helps explain the low status of medical microbiology. It may help to account for the neglect of Filipo Pacini's 1856 announcement of a vibrio associated with cholera, later belatedly named in his honor, *Vibrio cholerae*. Others too occasionally announced that they had discovered cholera's microbial cause. Their dismissal was usually both quick and contemptuous.

A second context was sensationalism, exploiting revulsion at the thought of microscopic life. Associated with dirt and decay, microbes were a proxy for impurity, and had publicity value. In the 1834 controversy over London's water supply, a few speculated that the recent cholera had been transmitted in Thames water contaminated with microscopic cholera-causing creatures. But the controversy was much more about monopoly than microbiology. The microscopist Arthur Hill Hassall reiterated the suggestion in 1850–1, when London's water was again under attack. The *Lancet* published his illustrations of the swarms of wee beasts (and fecal remains) in the waters that Londoners drank. Hassall too suspected a microbe to be the agent of cholera, but those he observed seemed too widely distributed to account for transitory outbreaks. Koch's critics would suggest that he should have emulated Hassall's caution; we now wonder that Hassall was not bolder. Even had he been, microscopy remained tainted by natural history.[2] As contributions to a controversy that had more to do with the water's price than its deadliness, such images of excremental life had some clout. Yet it is hard to escape the conclusion that good publicity came at the cost of scientific seriousness. The gullible masses might be swayed, but disgust should not move the intellect.

Quite different was an epidemiological and empirical contagionism, which avoided as far as possible the question of the identity of contagia. One found that each case had been in contact with a prior one. By some means, evidently, a body produced or reproduced an entity or influence able to trigger disease in another; one need not speculate what the agent was or how it did what it did. Thus smallpox: contact with a sufferer spread the disease; "lymph" from a pustule conferred immunity, but no one knew or needed to know what precisely changed bodies. The generic *virus* (not our "a virus") reflects those positivist commitments. So too (at least some of the time) would "germ" in the decades before "germ" would imply a species of bacterium. Both were placeholders: their opaqueness was a reminder that we knew not what they were, but only what they did. Solving practical problems of cholera control did not require knowing the nature of the contagion. Quarantine seemed warranted, but not for forty days. Goods did not transmit cholera, with the exception of personal linens.

These three perspectives are less schools than patterns of reasoning. In principle, the three are distinct: *either* cholera is a specific disease like smallpox, whether due to direct touch or to rare air; *or* it is just a bad griping of the guts. But, if the poles are clear, writers often are not; they are vague or varying in their use of terms. The phenomena of cholera are complicated. Each of the alternatives oversimplified or overlooked some facts. The very expectation of a single-factor explanation was, and is, unwarranted; we now recognize cholera as a product of multiple and interacting variables.

The special case of India

These were primarily European alternatives; beyond lies an Anglo-Indian positivism that is not French. Preoccupied with geographic and geophysical variables—winds, rains, temperatures, pressures, electrical states; also cholera's relation to drainage, altitude, soil type, and underlying bedrock—Anglo-Indian writers are often shunted into the anticontagionist catchall. But these factors figure differently: cholera is endemic in parts of India; it is, therefore, not aberrant but normal, and is to be understood as an element of place.

India owned the facts of cholera. As it approached Europe in the 1820s and 1830s, there was a premium for the export of those facts, and East India Company surgeons obliged with a spate of books. Their contents would be ore for rival theorists throughout the century. Usually the Anglo-Indians looked bemusedly on these theories —silly European speculations that would succumb to the next great bolus of Indian facts.

Owning data is a source of intellectual authority; one may ask, why the apparent reluctance to theorize? In Europe, theorizing about causes of cholera was taken up in the context of prevention. Writers may even defend theory choice in terms of hope. Thus contagionists argued that (some) anticontagionist theories (for example, those invoking epidemic constitution) undercut any hope of effective action. Better to act boldly if wrongly than to give in to calamity.

Where cholera was epidemic, an outrage, a violation of the normal, that approach makes sense. The European state could block its borders or ban pigs. But one does not remake the delta of the Bhramaputra or deflect the north-east monsoon. Cholera, the threatening enemy, may be spotted and perhaps stopped; cholera the norm is simply endured. The prospect is disturbing. The data-gathering Moloch of the meteorologically minded Anglo-Indians may seem an institution of well-researched fatalism. Hence, in a way that was not possible in Europe, cholera in India could be studied. An empirical science of cholera as a natural entity, as opposed to a series of half-baked attempts to manipulate it out of existence, is only possible once one has accepted it as something that must be accepted.

There was, in fact, an agenda. One did not stop cholera getting into India; it was already there. But one might get out of its way. Such mobility was the privilege of the colonizers. The East India Company's Army went where it would; the healthiest lands could be reserved for those it protected. Cholera writers, mostly regimental surgeons, focus on factors relevant to command. Their exemplar is neither the unremoved dung heap nor the diarrheal interloper crossing the border with sphincter tightly closed, but rather the commander who stops the cholera by shifting camp from valley bottom to airy hilltop (what Mary Lennox's frivolous parents, who stayed to party, should have done when cholera threatened).

Endemicity too could be a field for theory. If cholera is always potentially present, some factors must actualize its potential. Reginald Orton's massive *Essay on the Epidemic Cholera of India* (2nd edn, 1831) is the most sophisticated of the first generation of Indian cholera treatises. (I alluded to Orton's depression–decapitation analogy in the previous chapter.) Orton brings in a Galenic agenda of causal questions, draws from French physiology and a broad swathe of natural philosophy. He crosses categories. There is a "contagion" of cholera, a communicable organic poison, but he is more interested in its trigger—the "primary remote cause" in Galen's terms. This he takes to be low barometric pressure, linked in turn to atmospheric electro-negativity, minor variations in diurnal oxygen levels, and earthquakes.

To reach this conclusion, Orton drew on William Prout, H. B. de Saussure, Alessandro Volta, Humphry Davy, Joseph Priestley, Robert Boyle, Benjamin Franklin, James Hutton, Richard Kirwan, and especially Alexander von Humboldt, as well as a host of physicians and surgeons. He read volumes of travels, *The Encyclopedia Britannica*, and the Royal Society's *Philosophical Transactions*. He linked field to laboratory, and found a relevant experimental record in Boyle's air-pump experiments. Boyle had found that lowered air pressure induced vomiting, diarrhea, and convulsions, "*cholera*, in miniature."[3] The pestilence–earthquake link came from Noah Webster as a retrospective historical project. But there were now new variables—atmospheric electricity, the newly isolated gases, and caloric—that would make clear the underlying mechanisms.

Post-Koch, we have tended to see such extravagance in terms of red herrings and wild geese. The pages of hard-won data digested into tables and trends are empiricism run amok.

Projects like Orton's illustrate how desperate were the conceptual contortions to which cholera gave rise. Without sound theory, the mere collection of facts will as likely obscure as illuminate. Yet Orton's concern, cholera's periodicity, would be under-represented in the post-Snow, post-Koch paradigm. We still do not know what triggered the first pandemic or what periodically shakes cholera from its stupor and into an epidemic mode. The positivist may welcome open-ended empiricism; to dictate a priori which facts matter is to return to the web-spinning of earlier ages. And the Anglo-Indians were hardly equally open to all species of fact. Meteorology got more attention than demography.

Controversies, institutions, and genres

Reviewing the early nineteenth-century debates between contagionists and anticontagionists with regard to plague, yellow fever, and cholera, Erwin Ackerknecht held that, up to 1867, it would not have been possible to have made an evidence-based choice between the positions. By the end of the century things were clearer. Alternative hypotheses often reflected partial truths. Swamps and smells still mattered, but the "miasm" of malaria would be translated into its mosquito vectors, while cholera's miasm became a vibrio transmitted in crowded places without adequate excrement disposal. One might have anticipated this convergence; surely the proper attitude in such situations is patience and caution; research will sort things out in due course.

That did not happen. Early nineteenth-century cholera authors are known for impatience and unwarranted arrogance, rarely for humility and caution. Many are gratuitously dogmatic. They overstate, deny opposing evidence, use sloppy logic, browbeat. In the case of cholera, controversy persisted after 1867, even after 1884, when Koch isolated the cholera germ. Most believe it went on far too long: surely, after John Snow had shown cholera to be a fecal–oral disease transmissible by water, there were no grounds for anticontagionism. The patent relief of cholera historian Howard-Jones in narrating the suicide in 1901 of the Bavarian hygienist Max von Pettenkofer, seen as the great obfuscator, reflects a widely shared frustration.

Ackerknecht had suggested that, in the pre-1867 period, theory reflected ideology. Contagionism, implying quarantines and reflecting preoccupation with state security via border (and internal) surveillance, was the way of autocracy. Anticontagionism flourished in liberal states where there was faith in human betterment via representative institutions, in the free exchange of goods and ideas, and recognition of obligations to citizens. Given a lack of decisive evidence, ideology was a tie-breaker.

Contagionism and anticontagionism did dictate distinct and opposing cholera-prevention practices—in principle. If cholera spread person to person, it could be stopped by isolating the infected. If it were due to environmental and/or social conditions, these would need to be addressed. If you cannot act until you choose the right theory, there is incentive to make a best guess. Yet, as we have seen, those who actually managed the response to cholera did not find need for simple doctrines with clear and distinct implications. Many were happy eclectics. They adapted cholera practice—a mix of common sense, custom, hope, and affordability—from plague practice, itself eclectic. Moreover, most practices had more than one warrant: disinfection might neutralize contagia, destroy smell, or neutralize miasma.

But "just muddle through" will not do as public policy, however much it may describe reality. There were real policy issues—chiefly whether even to attempt quarantine—but the cholera debates were not shaped by practical needs, nor did they simply exhibit the hard and confusing work of induction.

We are stuck with a literature that frustrates. It is tendentious and facile. It is not that the books are wrong, but that authors could have done better with the materials at hand. As Howard-Jones complains, "contagionists and anti-contagionists made up their minds first and then selected the facts that seemed to fit their theories," as if anomalies would disappear if one pretended they did not exist.[4] They talk past one another, beg questions, misrepresent, demean, and even demonize. Plainly, this is not the international scientific community as we like to imagine it. Any blather about a brotherhood of inquirers is co-optive. That civility remains is surprising.

More than anything else, the debates reflect the imperative of immediacy. They manifest an ulterior ideology as well, in which problems—unruly facts no less than errant colleagues—are solved in print. Confusion is illusion; portending chaos will yield to the order of prose. One can write around anomalies and enigmas, and declare the proven routes to prevention and cure. It is the common concern with mastery that leads authors to discuss therapeutics jointly with etiology. There is no logical link; expertise in the one does not imply expertise in the other, yet these were the key sites of fear, the matters on which readers required resolution.

We still do this. We manage anxiety about looming environmental castastrophes on paper, justify egregious policies with paper trails that are presented as the fossil record of reason. Such means not only create authority to act but sustain the illusion that problems solved on paper no longer exist.

In what follows I focus on the comprehensive tracts and treatises. The large periodical literature on cholera represents undisciplined empiricism—authors report on the circumstances of local outbreaks and the results of therapies, but in this pre-paradigm period there is as yet no uniform language for observation and assessment. John Snow would draw on the periodical literature; many others ignored it.

Comprehensive works on cholera can be divided into three categories: (1) the exotics: works of European practitioners with experience in India or other parts of Asia; (2) reports to governments of quasi-official delegations sent to investigate epidemics foreign and domestic; (3) works for interested European and neo-European publics by those who fancied themselves cholera authorities.

The earliest of these genres consisted of the assessments of the "new disease" by Anglo-Indian military surgeons, considered above. These works began to appear in the mid 1820s; they are often the best early books on cholera; their authors—Annesley, Orton, Kennedy, even Ainslie, and earlier surgeons they drew on—were observant and experienced. Ostensibly, they wrote to establish a base line for regimental medical practice, but usually they did not address an exclusively medical audience. They generalized and speculated, but cautiously.

Fresh data from India were vital, but Anglo-Indian works did not carry European authority. Their books were tainted by the tropics, where diseases, and the persons getting them, were utterly other; and by the aura of professional inferiority that clung to anyone pursuing a medical career in such places (the best doctors, after all, ruled royal faculties or ancient hospitals and did not sail off to fever zones). Not only did the medical facts of India have no necessary bearing on civilized climes;

it was highly *unlikely* that illness in one was like illness in the other. That a distinct cholera spread from India to the rest of the world after 1817 was not an obvious inference; it defied what most expected.

Second, beginning in 1829, were the reports of expeditions to the cholera front lines, no longer far off in the Urals, but encroaching on European Russia. The delegates represented governments or medical academies, or sometimes just themselves. They were not cholera experts (the only experts were irredeemably Indian), but they were trusted advisers. Many were physicians of first rank. What they could expect to discover was how far this disease that threatened to spread to their own metropole was manageable. Were the peoples victimized by it like their own in race, liberty, and condition; were their doctors and quarantine enforcers competent, their hospitals adequate and well run? It was essential that each nation heard the news of cholera from reporters it trusted: the long history of plague diplomacy had been predicated on distrust of foreign medical misinformation. Even if there was no intent to deceive, standards, methods, statistics, and sensibilities in places like exotic Russia might differ from those in England, France, or Prussia.

Here too, there was no necessary premium on oversimplification. Manageability did not imply ability to cure or prevent. More important was reconciling expectations with reality. Only with sober knowledge of what was possible could a government keep order or a profession protect itself: for what better opportunity for the quacks was there than a new deadly and dreadful disease?

The third and the largest genre was the works of independent authors. It is here that the "why so many?" question arises. Just as nations required to hear the news of cholera from a trustworthy authority, so too were these authors each making a pitch to be taken as trusted translator to some imagined audience. To digest the mass of reports, transform confusion into confidence, was to declare to a community of readers one's status as their medical authority. These readers too are not mainly medical practitioners, though they are assumed to be well-enough versed in science and medicine to make some sense of cholera pathology. Mostly, readers are addressed as cholera citizens: in the private sphere, in civil society, even as executors of municipal or state responses to cholera, they will be taking decisions when the disease arrives.

The treatises were so many because the trust to which they appealed was essentially local. Authority came, not from what they knew of cholera, but from what readers knew of them; it was a matter of who they were, not what they knew. The Philadelphia society doctor Alfred Stillé was no cholera expert, but he was acknowledging Philadelphians' confidence in him. To present himself as writing only for Philadelphians would have been counter-productive. Medical authority was the union of universal knowledge with solicitous oversight of individuals; if non-Philadelphians were impressed by Stillé's insights, all the better. His city and his clients were surely fortunate to be attended by such a luminary.

The presumption of authors that they enjoy the trust of some readership is evident in the minimal pretence for writing they sometimes offer. The Glamorgan surgeon John Austin wrote in 1831, as cholera was threatening St Petersburg. His subtitle admits that his work will be derivative: *A Short and Faithful Account of the History, Progress, Causes, Symptoms, and Treatment of the Indian and Russian Cholera, taken from Authentic Sources, with Cases as Related by Practitioners in India.* Austin has never seen the Indian cholera, does not claim unusual skill in treating *cholera morbus.* Instead, on thirty years' experience as a surgeon, he will select statements "as appear to him...the most authentic."[5] Even the empiricist ethos of India did not prevent such pretense. He had never actually seen epidemic cholera, and it might seem "presumptuous" to write about it, Whitelaw Ainslie explained, but he had read Orton's book, and treated sporadic cholera.[6] Authors seem simultaneously to be saying, "I know nothing personally, and yet everything important." Such books are not necessarily bad; what is striking is the minimal ante required.

Logics and rhetoric

But the vast bulk of cholera treatises were, and still are, by private authors. Cholera was not really confusing, they often insist. It can be understood, prevented, and cured. But one's claim to such authority required driving from the field all claimants with incompatible ideas. Ironically, what made it confusing were the strident assertions that it was not. Many write against others. Nearly half of Hardin Weatherford's tiny 48-page *Treatise on Cholera, With the Causes, Symptoms, Mode of Prevention and Cure, on a New and Successful Plan* (Louisville, 1833) is an attack on another Louisville doctor who has put out a modest handbill on cholera prevention. Weatherford invites his nemesis to "guzzle [calomel] down his own throat, if he were taken with the Cholera!...I should, for one, say Good-bye, **most** respectable **DOCTOR**." He ends by declaring that "much learning" has made his adversary "mad," not simply wrong, and in need of "a straight jacket and confinement in a dark room."[7]

Why the iconoclasm?

The situation was desperate. Cholera came on; nothing worked. Modern science can be a cooperative endeavor because its practitioners trust in a shared training. Nineteenth-century cholera writers had much weaker ties of trust, and a correspondingly greater expectation that a single audacious sage could get it all right. Governments had an even greater need to create and project assurance. To a state, despotic or democratic, cholera was a problem of cosmic accountability. As a grave problem of theodicy, it called legitimacy into question: somehow, a sense had to be made of it, an adequate reason given for it. Less important than whether cholera was contagious or not was whether it could be brought within some plausible principle of order. Clarity, however contrived, was essential; confusion was disturbing as a sign of chaos, which was impermissible. That the experts did not subscribe to the same clarity was unfortunate, but it was much better that each had a clarity.

The best source of order was analogy. This apparently new disease had also to be rendered as not so very different from what God or nature regularly sent. The contagion–anticontagion structure had come down from the distant epidemic past. It offered well-defined templates in smallpox (plainly contagious) and intermittent fever–ague–malaria (apparently local). One had only to put cholera in the right box. And quickly. Cholera killed while fence-sitters waited for the facts to come in. No government would broadcast to its citizens that they were to be guinea pigs in the great cholera field trials, which would last until all its phenomena were fully revealed (its colonial subjects were another matter).

Does it matter that doctors, and states, so often changed their minds about causes and therapies? Hardly! Whatever experience led to, it was not humility. Writers were as sure in their new positions as they had been in their old. Rather, the ease with which minds changed indicates how little substance mattered.

Even in autocracies, action involved deliberation and required consent. To the bourgeois parliament of England no less than the Czar of all the Russias, what mattered was confidence: the enemy is familiar, there are means to vanquish him. To *change* policy was equally an assertion of confidence: we may not have known what we were doing before; now we do, and can go forth. A third possibility, that cholera is more different from, than similar to, the diseases we know, is disturbing. Departure from well-known tracks also requires confidence, and perhaps a willingness to relegate the cholera problem to the slow but certain process of scientific research.

The premiums on audacious authority, simplicity, and expediency within a context of decision-making bring to the fore debate as the primary idiom of cholera conversations. We do not look to debaters for tentativeness, self-criticism, or judicious, balanced appraisals. Their job, as the old song has it, is to accentuate the positive, eliminate the negative.

Recognizing the centrality of debate clarifies some features of the cholera literature, like the intoxication with dichotomy. Its great advantage was that evidence against one position was evidence for its opposite. With contagionism and anticontagionism defined as antitheses, a reasoner need only identify some putative implications of an opponent's supposed hypothesis, show these not to prevail, and QED. By the analogy of smallpox, contagionism implies that anyone exposed will take the disease. That does not happen. "Aha," shouts the inquirer (who, as author, knows how the story is to end)—the contagionist bogey is finally squashed.

Dichotomy exemplifies the most common attack tactic in these debates, the hypothetico-deductive trap. Hypothesizing was nearly unavoidable. Since key elements of the cholera process were inaccessible, it was necessary to deploy the "as if" of analogy. It was impossible to isolate *virus*, the contagionists' presumed agent, or to measure the precise state of atmosphere presumed to ignite cholera. And yet (as Orton exemplifies), the range of analogy is almost infinite, and in turn each can be plausibly linked to a wide range of consequences. One's own hypotheses were tentative and nuanced, sufficiently flexible to accommodate the confusing facts while the consequences of one's opponents' hypotheses were well defined and unfulfilled.

It is now clear—and the evidence was there in the nineteenth century—that cholera, like plague, and the many forms of "continued fever," including typhus and typhoid, did not readily fit into either box. And yet, against the comforting truth that whatever is "not A" must be "B," any third alternative is frightening in its sheer multidimensional indefiniteness. Even to entertain the possibility of a third box was to surrender to the trackless deserts of detail which would baffle every effort to produce comforting general laws of cholera.

Empiricism, however admirable, had little to commend it. The patterns apprehensible in the facts of cholera are many. Induction will require immersion in the dangerous waters of analogy. It will waste time and resources, and is no sure way to escape controversy. By contrast, to admit a finite, and small, list of possibilities and exclude all but one remains a common mode of medical reasoning. Much detail turns out to be incidental; "simplest first" is an economical decision theory. Early nineteenth-century systems of pathology and therapeutics embodied such practices; many were built on dichotomy. Most medicines were either to strengthen the debilitated body or to calm the overstimulated one.

The power of dichotomy is evident in the asymmetry of contagionism–anticontagionism. Even if contagion may be—though rarely was—a clear and distinct idea, we have no right to expect coherence from the catchall of anticontagionism, defined as a negative. Who benefited from that asymmetry depended on the allocation of burden of proof. Infused with revolutionary positivism, early nineteenth-century French clinicians found anticontagionism a rubric for emphasizing how much was not not known. Facts could be assembled, but theoretical entities like "contagia" were speculations. On the other hand, if anticontagionism could be made into a position, rather than the absence of one, it could be rejected as arbitrary, imprecise, even tautological: "cholera happened when its cause was present." Either the claim was untestable, hence unscientific, or, if testable (as when some aerial poison, like hydrogen sulfide, was posited as the cause of cholera), then shown as wrong. Either the presence of the suspect agent did not always generate cholera, or cholera occurred without it, or whatever it did to an animal was not really cholera at all. Oversimplification was not invariably a refuter's tool; for both sides oversimplification of their own views—for example, Edwin Chadwick's mantra, of all smell as disease—might serve particular rhetorical needs.

In fact there was a third option: a specific agent mediated by environmental and social factors. This "contingent contagionism" was considered in 1832 but dropped out of sight, though it would be an increasingly accurate label for positions writers actually held, as opposed to those ascribed to them. But, for public purposes, the antinomies were useful, if only to refute the supposed oversimplifications of others.

Facts and narratives

Even where there was experience, it was so easy to go beyond it. Nelson, writing in 1866, was insistent that his book, unlike so many others, would represent personal experience (he had been medical officer in Montreal during 1832–4). But Nelson, like so many others, was quick to overstate. Cholera "never, in a single instance, preceded the arrival of affected persons or things," he declared. It struck with equal severity, regardless of place, race, climate, poverty, or sanitary condition. One single case, the outbreak in the harem at Shiraz, proved the impotence even of "extreme cleanliness and hygiene." Nelson simply ignored amassed data showing that cholera did not spread everywhere, nor evenly in any community. Those who disagree (including Anglo-Indian cholera writers) are demented: a "disgrace of human understanding." Nelson was fiercest on therapeutics. One might expect his caustic review of the extreme remedies derived from arbitrary and opposite pathologies to preface a call for lowered expectations and more research. The parody-satire simply introduces Nelson's own cholera cure.[8] Nelson's book is far better than Weatherford's tirade. He is experienced, well read, insightful, accurate. Yet his posture to readers and colleagues—doughty defense of empiricism in service of dogma—precludes any real empiricism.

Yet, even when the facts were on the table, they might be read oppositely. The contrast with the post-watershed cholera literature, in which multiple explanations are kept in consideration as long as possible, and conclusions are often advanced not merely tentatively, but apologetically, is striking. Seemingly empirical questions were vested in rival stories in which the glass was either half empty or half full. These were stories about whether doctors and nurses got cholera, whether it spread in and from ships, and about whether every outbreak could be traced to a previous outbreak.

The relative vulnerability of doctors and nurses in cholera hospitals, surely a matter of fact, was the subject of one of the longest battles. It was an issue in 1830 and still one in 1890. At first it seemed that Russian doctors did not get cholera; this, more than the ineffectiveness of cordons, was reason to abandon efforts to isolate. When some did get it, the contagionists' stock rose, if briefly. In outbreak after outbreak, hospital staff were stricken disproportionately more often than the population at large (depending on how large that reference population was conceived to be), but at a much lower rate than in (contagious) typhus. Cholera was simultaneously more contagious than a non-contagious disease and less contagious than a contagious one. And, even if doctors did get it unduly, that proved nothing: unless supremely well ventilated, a cholera hospital would generate its own local miasm.

Similarly with the cholera swallowers. Cholera had more than its share of auto-experimenters, who would gulp down comma bacillus cultures or other extracts of cholera excretion to prove their claims of harmlessness (thus putting their mouths were their money was). Howard-Jones reports twenty-seven in all, none of whom came down with cholera. Best known was Max von Pettenkofer, who in 1892 swallowed a cubic centimeter of culture (having first neutralized his stomach to allow the microbe safe passage to its site of supposed operation in the upper bowel). The experiments were to refute contagion. But who bore the burden of proof? If only one subject sickened, insisted contagionists, that proved contagion. If none did, that did not disprove it: surely no one expected every contact with contagion to induce disease—unless, that is, one used the analogy of smallpox. Or the experiments showed nothing, since even a positive result could be ascribed to incidental factors. Ironically, these overwhelmingly negative results have come down to us as positive, on the basis of the case of Rudolph Emmerich, a Pettenkoferian who did get a significant diarrhea (and sometimes, erroneously, is even said to have died from it).

UN DOCTEUR ÉPATANT

POUR PROUVER QUE LE CHOLÉRA N'EST PAS CONTAGIEUX
le docteur N... se fourre une déjection de cholérique par la bouche; — cinq minutes après, il rend un bouquet de violettes par... autre part.

10. Max von Petteknkofer was only the best known of a parade of cholera swallowers, each hoping to prove in the most graphic way that cholera was not contagious. This 1884 French cartoon may refer to Bochefontaine's 1884 ingestion. (*Visages du Cholera*)

Surely, if cholera persisted on a ship passing through many climes and then appeared on a remote island following the arrival of that ship, it could not be a function of locale, and must be contagious! The 1819 epidemic on the Indian Ocean island of Mauritius was proof enough for Bisset Hawkins and Gilbert Blane. Here, too, facts had to be judged against expectations, which were fungible. And there were instances in which cholera broke out as a ship neared land. It was more a disease of the harbor than of the open ocean. That suggested that its agent— if there was one—could not long maintain itself away from its home. And, of course, a ship was itself an environment.

And, finally, there was general claim that every case could be attributed to a prior case: to the arrival of a victim or an infected article, usually clothing or bedding. How hard it is to find such an index case depends on what counts as proof. Contagionists lowered the bar, non-contagionists raised it. In the 1883 Darmietta outbreak in Egypt, English investigators exonerated those suspected of introducing the disease. To no avail: the Nile delta was in regular contact with choleraic Mumbai. If these persons had not brought the disease, someone else surely had. Since British captains were known to be duplicitous and greedy and British port authorities lax, the finding by British epidemiologists of no evidence of transmission constituted evidence of transmission.

And now Dr Snow

Only in light of this complexity can we make sense of John Snow. He is cholera's cult figure, hero in the legend of the Broad Street pump (of the removal of the pump handle, following Snow's proof that its water had spread cholera in one London neighborhood). He is far better known now than he was in his lifetime. It is he who painstakingly follows facts and battles complacency and obscurantism. He gets so many things right that others have looked either venal or subnormal by comparison.

In 1849 Dr Snow was an upwardly mobile Yorkshireman with a modest practice, bootstrapping his way into London's medico-scientific circles through research on the inhalation of anesthetic gases. In that year appeared the first edition of his pamphlet "On the Mode of Communication of Cholera." In this first (32-page) edition of the pamphlet Snow asserted the *communicability* of cholera (not, notably, its *contagiousness*), chiefly on the basis of a number of (English) cases in which outbreaks had apparently followed contamination of a water supply by the excrement of a cholera sufferer. The review is impressive, but the evidence is selected; the essay does not stand out from the works of others who used similar methods to make the case for other variables.

The second edition (January 1855) was three times longer, bolstered by two complementary "natural experiments," occurring during the London cholera of 1853–4. First was a comparative analysis of cholera mortality in the districts served by two south London water companies. The Lambeth used a relatively purer upstream source, the Southwark and Vauxhall still drew its water from the sewer-lined tidal Thames. In earlier decades these companies had competed in a portion of their respective districts. Mains from both ran beneath some streets; adjacent houses might be served by different companies. In such districts, it would seem that every variable but water would have been randomized. Cholera deaths per household (for the companies' service districts overall) differed by roughly an order of magnitude. Initially it proved difficult to narrow the focus to the areas of entangled mains; that problem would be largely resolved in the following year (though Snow is best known for "Mode of Communication," follow-up articles extended his argument in important ways).

Second was the Golden Square mini-epidemic. At the end of August 1854 cholera erupted in a single Soho neighborhood, killing more than 500 in a little over a week. Snow found that use of water from a pump in Broad Street was a common factor. He showed further that two relatively cholera-free populations near the pump—workers at a brewery and residents of a workhouse—had their own wells. And, finally, he showed that some cholera cases far from the pump had used its water. Best known is the "Hampstead widow," who received her favorite water from visiting relatives. These last facts clinch: the distribution of cholera around the well is suggestive; even more so is the fact that victims actually used the water. Any remaining doubt should dissolve when anomalies—the uneven distribution of the disease concentrically around the well—not only fall within the theory but become evidence for it. For Snow, these natural experiments refute the claim that cholera is a function of place alone, and demonstrate instead that water is the key determinant.

How had Snow come to focus on water? The hypothesis that cholera was communicable was widely held; why go further to posit an ingested agent and a waterborne one at that? Others who believed in a cholera contagion either saw no need to identify a particular point of entry or, evidently, assumed that it was inhaled.

None of the usual explanations is wholly satisfactory. One is that Snow was testing an induction. Perhaps he had noted, in a careful reading of the cholera literature, the frequent

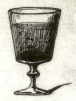

This is the water that JOHN drinks.

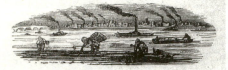

This is the Thames with its cento of stink,
That supplies the water that JOHN drinks.

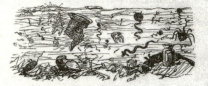

These are the fish that float in the ink-
-y stream of the Thames with its cento of stink,
That supplies the water that JOHN drinks

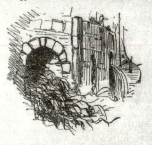

This is the sewer, from cesspool and sink,
That feeds the fish that float in the ink-
-y stream of the Thames with its cento of stink,
That supplies the water that JOHN drinks.

11. John Snow is known for bringing attention to the danger of contaminated drinking water. But such waters were repellent before his great insights, as in this 1849 Punch cartoon here, nor did his demonstrations bring quick changes. (*Wellcome Library, London*)

CHOLERA

AND

WATER.

BOARD OF WORKS

FOR THE LIMEHOUSE DISTRICT,

Comprising Limehouse, Ratcliff, Shadwell, and Wapping.

The INHABITANTS of the District within which CHOLERA IS PREVAILING, are earnestly advised

NOT TO DRINK ANY WATER WHICH HAS NOT PREVIOUSLY BEEN BOILED.

Fresh Water ought to be Boiled every Morning for the day's use, and what remains of it ought to be thrown away at night. The Water ought not to stand where any kind of dirt can get into it, and great care ought to be given to see that Water Butts and Cisterns are free from dirt.

BY ORDER,

THOS. W. RATCLIFF,
CLERK OF THE BOARD.

Board Offices, White Horse Street,
1st August, 1866.

12. This 1866 East London cholera poster was more effective in spurring change. (*Wellcome Library, London*)

concurrence of cholera with contaminated water. Yet, despite Snow's list of cases, few accounts of local cholera paid much attention to water quality; the facts were not there to mount the inference. Or Snow's focus on water might be seen in terms of the campaign for reform of London's water supply. Several schemes had been proposed in 1848–50. Thames water was accused of harming health, even of causing cholera, but economic and ideological issues were more important: water was a right not a costly commodity. Snow's findings in 1854 (three years after the reform movement had collapsed into the compromise Metropolitan Water Act of 1851) would be fuel for later water reformers, yet, unlike his colleague Arthur Hassall, he does not seem to have been a partisan in 1850. He was more concerned with the sewer-building that had contaminated the river, though it is not clear what alternative he would propose to the new water closet.

Snow's own explanation—that he fixed on an ingestible agent because cholera's first symptoms were gastrointestinal—simply relocates the question. Snow views cholera as an irritation of the lining of the bowel. Many did not see it as localized. Its diarrhea might be incidental: it was not invariably the first symptom, did not occur in all cases. Nor did most physicians accept that symptoms in the guts implied an oral agent.

To seek a single starting point may be misconceived. For what has struck many about Snow's cholera theory is the reciprocity of epidemiology and pathology. Before taking up cholera, Snow had studied anesthetics; he was one of the few cholera writers able to move easily between pathophysiology and epidemiology. During his years of cholera research, he was thinking about the characteristics of the special "morbid poisons" of diseases in both contexts. As much as anything, the logic may have been one of exclusion: gripings of the gut may not imply oral intake, yet the poison must enter and the gas laws suggest inhalation of a concentrated poison to be unlikely—at least to Snow. The gas laws were *ideal* after all, and others hypothesized entities akin to aerosols. Other features must be explained—how the poison might exit the body in sufficient quantity and concentration to initiate new cases. A candidate for the simultaneous solution of these several problems is a fecal–oral, waterborne, organic (quasi-biological, self-replicating) agent. Other models may fit; and we must keep in mind that for Snow—not always for his disciples—water is not the necessary means of cholera transmission, but the actual one in London.

Snow's work was noticed and appreciated. It was seen to demonstrate that bad water was probably a factor in cholera, perhaps an important one. But it was folded into the mix; it complemented rather than replaced. His colleagues' failure to see genius in their midst has been attributed to bias; lost in their own miasmatic fog, they could neither see fact nor follow reason. Such assessments are unhelpful. We need to see how Snow, though an "honest and conscientious observer" of unsurpassed "diligence," might have been "biased by his creed."[9]

These are the words of E. A. Parkes, an exacting yet respectful critic. Parkes, like Snow, was both pathologist and epidemiologist. Six years younger than Snow, he was a success: professor at University College, editor of a major journal, already with extensive cholera experience in India and Crimea. As author of the best-known manual of sanitary science, Parkes would become, with John Simon, one of the architects of mid-Victorian contingent-contagionism.

Parkes does not push his own cholera views; rather, he evaluates each of Snow's claims, though serially rather than collectively. His is a devil's advocacy, a classic instance of the scientific virtue of organized skepticism. Sometimes he under-appreciates, but generally his assessment is fair. Parkes admits a prima facie case against water—enough for indictment but not conviction. Apparently water has an important role in some cholera, but not to the exclusion of other factors. Snow could have done more to convince, but Parkes doubts further inquiry would confirm Snow's claims. Parkes helps us appreciate why mid-nineteenth-century epidemiology was so hard and why cholera was genuinely confusing. Not all his criticisms could be met; together they show us where Snow had overstretched and why others were reluctant to go along.

Parkes notes that Snow's epidemiology is uneven. Seeking to link cholera with water, he sometimes uses raw numbers of cholera victims rather than ratios, and uses households, streets, or districts, not population, as a denominator. Sometimes Snow was simply borrowing incomplete results from others, but at other times he seems oblivious to the importance of the denom-inator. Parkes complains that Snow was also uninterested in fac-tors other than water, like age, occupation, or habit (he leaves out sex).[10] In the Broad Street case, so too in south London, Snow had *argued* that other factors were not significant rather than *showing* that they were not. In the former, he had shown that drinking pump water was a common element among those who got cholera. He had also shown that, in two discrete popu-lations, non-use of this water was a common element among non-sufferers. He had, he thought, excluded the possibility that cholera incidence was simply spatial, but he had not thoroughly explored other variables. He did not worry about the propor-tion of all users who took cholera, or the proportion of all non-users who did not, both of which would have been important in comparing the power of Broad Street pump water against other variables. (Revd Henry Whitehead, a local curate who supplemented Snow's study, did try to gauge the proportion of users who got cholera, but only for part of the area.)

Parkes also questioned those prize facts that clinch the case for Snow—the Hampstead widow, struck by cholera despite living far from the Broad Street well: "unanswerable," if correct (even more telling was her Islington niece, who got cholera from taking the water onward). But is this a single datum or a crucial experiment? For Snow, the power of the case was commensurate to its unexpectedness: the Broad Street outbreak might be a story of water and place; this was one of water alone. Yet the argument was *post hoc, propter hoc* as Parkes pointed out, using another Snow example—of a landlord, trying to convince a surveyor of the safety of the water in houses he rents, who drinks the water and dies of cholera. This, to Parkes, smacks of coincidence. On such grounds, any antecedent can be cause. Do *all* distant Broad Street pump-users get cholera? Snow does not know. Do *all* distant cholera cases drink Broad Street water? He does not so claim. Had the widow been subject to other choleragenic influences? Snow assumes not, but cannot know. Coincidences abound in large populations. To find a hypothesis-confirming link does not rule out other links that one has not sought. Both Parkes, and later Max von Pettenkofer, who repeats the charge, are groping toward what would now be called a case-control study of risk factors. Would Broad Street pump water jump out in such an analysis? Only if one set spatial and temporal boundaries and chose variables appropriately.

Parkes worries that there is no independent analytical corroboration for Snow's inference, nor any candidate pathogen. Snow does not know that the Broad Street pump had been contaminated, or with what. Rather, he assumes entities and events on the basis of the results they would presumably produce. In positing an unidentified morbid poison, he was doing nothing others were not also doing, but, in the case of Broad Street, Snow was forced to defy both chemistry and microscopy. Neither method disclosed anything unusual that might stand as a choleragen; moreover, the Broad Street water was apparently purer than waters that did not cause cholera. In this instance Snow would be vindicated in letting epidemiological inferences trump analytical facts, yet the rule is not a general one, nor did Snow follow it uniformly: he invokes negative analytical evidence in excluding air. Followers of Koch would declare that cholera-like diarrheal disease in the absence of *Vibrio cholerae* was not cholera; analysis would trump epidemiology. If any measureable condition of water can be compatible with any claim about its tendency to cause cholera, Parkes argues that Snow's hypothesis can never be tested. Nor is Snow concerned about a form of corroboration that would become central—the index case, the finding of the one whose bowels had done the dirty deed. He could say *when* contamination of the Broad Street pump had occurred; again, Whitehead would identify a probable first case (of infant diarrhea, not cholera). The absence of a candidate cholera agent did not bother Parkes unduly; it did lead others, particularly William Budd, to hesitate. Budd would not claim waterborne transmission until he could say what precisely was being transmitted.

Snow made correlation not only into causation, but into mono-causation. In elevating water he ignored other factors: indeed, the case for water became a case against them. His move embodies three assumptions: that cholera is a specific disease entity; that it is the exclusive product of a unique agent rather than the vector sum of pathological forces; and that the agent has only one way into the body. Many saw no reason to adopt any of these; at the time, they were less testable hypotheses than metaphysical positions. The assumption that like effects even imply like causes was not universally held: any clinician knew that common symptoms could have quite different causes. Within such a framework it was easy to see the role of water as predisposing only.

Parkes worried that Snow might have set a higher burden of proof than he could meet. "He has not been able to prove that all were attacked who drank this water, and that none were attacked who did not drink."[11] In South London, only a small proportion of those presumably exposed were attacked; the proportion was (probably) larger on Broad Street, but, since anyone could use the well, Snow could not say precisely; there is no way to fix an exact denominator. But did he have to? If cholera were the product of multiple and differing causes, the variability of its incidence was unproblematic. But Snow, with many younger Paris-influenced physicians, was drawn to a toxicological model. The cholera poison irritated the lining of the gut. Its effects resembled those of mineral and organic poisons. Yet the more precisely one conceptualized such poisons, the greater the problem of their occasional (or frequent) inaction. One could— Snow did—propose that the cholera poison was not uniformly distributed: it might be particulate, a phenomenon of natural history not chemistry. A critical mass might be necessary. At the time, the assumptions were gratuitous. Snow did not seek to test them, for example, by correlating the amount of water one drank with the likelihood of cholera.

Most importantly, Snow universalized, moving from demonstrating an important role for water in some outbreaks to cholera as waterborne disease, and not only cholera but probably yellow fever, malaria, and plague, as well as typhoid fever. It would be more correct, Richard Feachum has pointed out, to see Snow as articulator of a concept of fecal–oral disease. He argued that, while unhygienic defecation habits might account for the spread of cholera within a family, only contaminated water could account for its explosive impact on a town: Parkes was correct, but misleading, when he ascribed to Snow the view that cholera was "propagated" exclusively by water.[12]

Is Snow, as is often suggested, the consummate reasoner? He is systematic and painstaking; he thinks on many levels. And lucky: his ad hoc explanations and assumptions about inaccessibles turn out largely to have been right. And yet his success, like Koch's later, came from paying not more attention to the facts, but less. It may well sometimes be best to ignore complexity, forestall the wet-blanket metaphysicians with their kvetching about unwarranted inferences, and leap into a "what if" mode. Anomalies will be resolved; until they are, best to push on in heady oversimplification. Parkes rightly treats Snow's achievement as neither proof nor induction, but as argument. Snow marshals evidence to support a hypothesis that pre-existed the gathering of facts. Enter Snow's universe, and all makes sense, but nothing compels entry. Neither in style nor in substance did that argument stand out from the partisan cholera literature of preceding decades, even if it did so in quality.

Hence Parkes's strategy of restraint and assimilation. Snow is on to something. Toned down, his findings will take their place in cholera science. But he overreaches. A petit bourgeois from York, he is naive—a nice man who knows not what he is up against. He has ignored or alienated the sanitarians; failed to gain a hospital professorship or public-health post. A theory like Snow's must be promoted. Snow tried, but died in 1858. When Koch took up the campaign thirty years later, he did so as developer of a powerful new methodology and from a position of institutional power, and still had to battle to convince colleagues.

Parkes had been right to worry. Relatively quickly Snow's work vanished into the black hole that swallowed cholera publications. Rejuvenated by William Farr and Edward Frankland following the London cholera of 1866, the cholera–water link lived on, often attributed to these or others, even to the chief medical officer John Simon, who in 1855–6 had rejected Snow's conclusion while appropriating his demonstration (linking cholera to water source in south London).

Yet there was gradual convergence around the idea that cholera was a fecal (or "filth") disease, caused by a specific agent. Urban filth in general became a lesser concern than human excrement, and especially human excrement during cholera outbreaks. There seemed no reason to restrict "fecal" to "fecal–oral" or to focus exclusively on water. It might be the main means of cholera transmission in London and in a handful of other major urban outbreaks, but many towns hard hit by cholera did not have piped water from central sources.

Caution and inclusion dominated English public health in the post-Snow years. The diplomatic John Simon had replaced the doctrinaire Edwin Chadwick. Simon, with the like-minded Parkes and William Farr, pursued a policy of broadly based sanitary reform and long-term epidemiological and pathological research. In the case of cholera, that research might be a way beyond shrill denunciation.

Beyond Snow

Snow was a powerful reasoner. Others were too. They weighed the facts differently. As statistician to England's Registrar General for Births, Deaths, and Marriages, the Paris-trained Farr was well placed to order the incoming cholera data. Using the records for the 1849 epidemic, Farr studied the relation of cholera mortality to elevation. With regard to England overall, cholera was a disease of valleys and coasts: mortality per capita was three times higher on the coasts. If one focused on the great towns, cholera struck much more heavily in ports than in inland manufacturing towns, even though population was denser in the latter. That relation did not hold for mortality overall, nor for diarrheal mortality. In London, cholera was a riverside killer; mortality dropped off as one moved up the London basin—so steadily that Farr could write an equation for the curve. The Indian data fit: Bengal, after all, was low; cholera was less prevalent in the Himalayan foothills.

Farr held that, for London, elevation was a better predictor of cholera mortality "than any other known element." He could compare variables individually, but the mathematics did not exist to disentangle the effect of one variable from others with which it was partially concurrent. He considered wealth, population density, and persons/household. But, while "the effects of the water and…wealth…are apparent, they do not…conceal the effects of elevation." In the early 1880s, Berlin's August Hirsch, omni-expert on infectious disease, would see the elevation law as the greatest empirical generalization on cholera.

Farr would help Snow with statistics on the south London water fields, but, unlike Snow, he was not hoping to disclose a single factor. Foremost a statistician, Farr was interested in other variables: season, precipitation, wind, temperature. These, like elevation, were akin to what we would call risk factors. Even if he saw no ready way to integrate these, he was wedded to the idea of composite causation. He was not uninterested in necessary specific agents. The law of elevation suggested an environmental explanation for their operation. Decomposing matter would accumulate in low-lying places. Cholera depended on the quantity of such matter, but even more on "some *change* in … [its] *chemical action*."[13]

Henry Acland did find the 1854 cholera to be waterborne, but not exclusively. The 317 cases of cholera or choleraic diarrhea in Oxford and surrounding villages represented a series of mini-outbreaks. One of these was in the county gaol. Water was suspected and the supply changed. There had been twenty-five cases before the change; there were only four mild cases after it. Acland, who knew of Snow's work, concluded: "We cannot reasonably doubt the immediate connection between the Water and the existence of the Disease, nor question the cause of its cessation in this particular instance."[14]

Acland has confirmed Snow—and more. If one suspects x to cause y, y should stop when x stops. The Broad Street pump's handle had been removed, but only after the Soho epidemic had virtually ended. And a gaol was a better experimental setting: nutrition, occupation, and sanitation were constant, the water supply alone had changed. Confirmation came in the form of the case of a laundress who had taken in linens and clothes of a cholera victim. To keep her from washing them, her terrified neighbors (more likely to have been expressing lay contagionism than to have read John Snow) took away the pump handle and burned some of the clothing. Another laundress took the rest. She came down with cholera and spread it to her family.

That a water–cholera link was sometimes clear (Acland praised Snow) did not warrant seeing the Oxford outbreak as being due to a single cause. After discussing the gaol outbreak, Acland moves on to pages of statistics on ozone levels. These, not water, might explain the cholera among agricultural laborers in outlying villages. Hidden contacts might also explain such isolated cases, but in Acland's view we had no business reading negative evidence as positive. Cholera may sometimes be spontaneous. Acland's atmospheric anomalies may be equally ad hoc, yet the atmosphere, an entity existing everywhere but everywhere different, seems a good place to look. And there are newly recognized variables that can plausibly be linked to cholera. Electrical states had excited Orton; the new ozone intrigued Acland.

His was a very tentative theory: atmospheric states caused diarrhea, which then, in some cases, produced the transmissible cholera poison. This could spread in air or water, take root in lungs or in gut. Each outbreak would exhibit a unique mix of means of transmission/causation. Everywhere it made sense to disinfect cholera evacuations and purify sewage. Acland's emergent contagion view validates a question in answering it: the question of the origin of epidemics, one that Snow sidesteps.

Like Parkes and Farr, Acland is uneasy with attempts like Snow's to simplify by concentrating on outbreaks that most clearly reflect a favored factor. Better to keep all the facts of cholera before one, and all options under consideration *as long as possible*. With the facts thus corralled, truth may be squeezed out by gradually tightening that ring. But one must guard against oversimplification. Extrapolating from some cholera to all was what had led to the acrimonious debates between contagionists and anticontagionists. The view that impure water was a factor, but that it operated only by predisposition, dispensed with the need to find a cholera agent—William Budd's concern. Evidence linking cholera to water could be included; evidence linking it to other factors need not be excluded—a prudent and diplomatic, if not an adventurous stance.

What difference would it have made had Snow's contemporaries interpreted his findings as we do? The movement to improve London's water had already begun; it would putter on. Cholera worries had not been, nor would they be, the main issue. Nor was (or is) cholera prevention obviously the responsibility of the vendor of a cholera-spreading medium, however much we might wish it were so. Given the continued occurrence of waterborne diseases in a world that sees Snow as right, it is plain that his truths have not been sufficient imperative for safe water for all. Finally, to the degree that focus on water might have allowed neglect of other social and environmental improvement, the prospect is problematic. Snow's 1855 testimony in support of "noxious trades" has disturbed: logically, recognition of specific agents does not entail an exoneration of chronic assaults on health; it did for Snow. An Aclandesque public health based in community development finds room for both.

Pax zymotica, 1860–1885

The decades that separated Snow from Koch reveal grudging convergence in theory and in practice, precisely the squeezing of facts I have alluded to. Controversy persists. If no less acrimonious, it is generally more civil, reined in by the International Sanitary Conferences. Their determinations lacked teeth, but, in defining the center of opinion, they put pressure on those like the contrarian British, with their extreme view that cholera was local eruption not communicable disease. Most held that cholera was a specific disease caused by a specific agent. Whether the agent need always have come from a previous victim was unclear.

In science, as in diplomacy, creative ambiguity can calm fruitless conflict. In the case of cholera, that calm came from the zymotic concept, an old idea, rehabilitated and made a central element of organic chemistry by the German chemist Justus Liebig, further transformed into a deep theory of pathology by William Farr, both in the early 1840s. As understood by Liebig, large organic molecules—like those of living beings—decomposed in distinct ways upon contact with other large organic molecules decomposing in those ways. That distinctiveness was understood to be kinetic, a distinct form of shaking apart. Such decomposition came under the general heading of fermentation. It could be posited that each of the filth-related diseases represented a species of fermentation. Farr proposed to call the ferment of each disease its "zyme," just as we speak of its germ.

Such zymes might affect the guts, nerves, or lungs; they might come in through air, water, or across the skin. Conferred to susceptible tissues or fluids of the body, this zymotic process would account for the pathological changes specific to the disease. Returned to air, water, or soil in the excreta of the victim, the ferment might pass directly to new victims or propagate further in some susceptible organic "nidus" such as sewage, water, or filthy soil. As Alexander Wynter Blyth explained it: "If we were to suppose a seed of disease planted in a rich, fertile soil of decomposing matter, we should give a pretty fair description of the fostering effect of impurity on disease. It would, in fact, appear as if the putrid matter itself took the disease and passed it to the living."[15] Zymotic diseases were communicable, but not necessarily exclusively: the distinct decomposition might generate spontaneously.

Snow himself developed a version of the concept in his most obscure work, an 1852 address "On the Mode of Continuous Molecular Changes."[16] The essay—scholastic in its abstractness and qualification—is not explicitly about cholera, but in it Snow creates a framework of plausibility that will unite his epidemiology and pathology. Snow's argument, like Liebig's and Farr's, is that a large class of phenomena may be understood as the transmission of modes of molecular change. These include contagious diseases (a sufferer transmits a mode of pathological change to a new victim), life itself (reproduction is transmission of organic processes), organic decomposition (rot spreads in susceptible matters), and some inorganic processes.

This analogical framework will allow Snow to entertain a germ theory of disease. Perhaps contagion or rot act as they do as attributes of living things, which also act that way. It may be fruitful to pursue the analogy that contagia are alive, but Snow stops short of claiming that they do what they do *because* they are alive. That move would be from lesser to greater obscurity. For Snow, "molecular changes" allowed access to the specificity the germ theory would bring, but in a way that insulated such consideration from the complaint that *contagium animatum* was an ad hoc explanation, and equally from the limitations of microscopy. Contagious capability need not be housed in a life form; whether it is, or what one means by "life" and "living" at this microscopic level, is moot. One presumes simply that chemistry explains things in a way that any merely vital process cannot; at bottom, any pathological process is a chemical one. A century later, recognition of the operation of the cholera toxin would fulfill the quest. Snow's conception of cholera did not require "molecular changes," yet such zymotic deep theory provided coherence and hence credibility for his other inferences.

It did so for others too. More metaphor than theory, "zymotic" illuminated without restricting. There were *no ways* of independently measuring the distinct kinetic states of the decomposing filth other than by the diseases it caused, hence no testable consequences. A single modest experiment was given undue importance. Karl Thiersch had shown in 1856 that mice were killed by ingesting bits of paper saturated in cholera excreta, but only after the paper had festered for a few days: fresh excreta had no effect. Confirmed by John Burdon-Sanderson, the experiment was the zymoticists' paradigm exemplar.

The metaphor was a fertile one; it put Louis Pasteur on a course of research that would equate the chemical change of each fermentation with a species of microbe—first for fermentations producing beer, wine, and vinegar, then for the "diseases" that sometimes spoiled these products, and ultimately for the diseases of animals and humans. The equation of fermentation to species brought great advantages: the microbe of each disease might be recognized; the conditions of its existence worked out, and means taken for its destruction. Once crossed, the zymotic bridge from pathology to etiology was no longer needed. The Prussian country doctor Robert Koch was concerned simply with tracking down disease germs. Koch's way was both scientific and practical: there were innumerable germs to be found; being finally able to see what they were hunting, public officers could act with precision. If germs could be destroyed, pathology, and therapeutics too, became redundant.

As a form of contingent contagionism, zymotic theory combined the contagionists' conviction of communicability with the sanitarians' focus on filth. An ancient and respected *explanandum*, fermentation and disease had been linked long before Liebig. However flexible, the metaphor still implied practical steps: removal of filth, isolation of victims, and disinfection of their excreta. The old concern with predisposing causes could be maintained. Strong and healthy tissues and fluids resisted zymotic disturbance; hunger, with a debilitating environment generally, contributed to cholera. Not only did zymotic theory skirt unanswerable questions about the nature and actions of the agent; other vexed questions receded too. The origin of pandemics, Orton's question, became an antiquarian matter, pushed beyond contingency to mere randomness.

One should not overstate; the "peace" was relative. Writers continued to complain of "vigorous intolerance," even as they perpetuated it. The periodicity and geography of outbreaks remained controversial.

The impresario of this *pax cholera* was the Bavarian hygienist Max von Pettenkofer (1818–1901). Pettenkofer's reputation, too, is the product of myth-making; he is villain in a historiography dominated by Snow and Koch. He refused to see cholera as waterborne and defied the bacteriological gospel, holding to increasingly obsolete sanitarian dogma. His English-language biographer, Edgar Hume, could say only that he had "stimulated others"—to refute his errors. Worse, he is said to have seduced many: John Simon, England's influential medical officer during the 1860s and early 1870s, and his successors are often seen as Pettenkoferians, as are the leading Anglo-Indian medics (actually, they had considered but rejected Pettenkofer's theories—he was but another imperious European). In fact, in broad focus, his views were generic among zymoticists.

Pettenkofer's career moved across chemistry, human physiology, general matters of urban hygiene, and on to cholera.

Winning the support of the King of Bavaria, he was well positioned, as journal editor and institute head, to promote a research agenda and establish a clearing-house for cholera data. His first cholera publication was in 1855, the year of Snow's triumph.

His ideas are hard to pin down, in part because they evolved. Most familiar are the xyz model and the ground-water hypothesis. The former approaches truism, but would distinguish Pettenkofer's view from that of post-Koch theorists. z is the specific poison or the proximate cause of cholera; it depends on x, a specific agent, and y, a set of contributing conditions. y could include both internal factors of predisposition within a population and external conditions affecting the agent. Pettenkofer would come to accept Koch's comma bacillus as x, but the actual poison of cholera was not it but something it somehow helped to engender in certain conditions. There is an analogy to the later concept of a cholera toxin, but in Pettenkofer's version the toxin is emitted outside the body and acts independently from the entity that has produced it—imagine a ptomaine wafting up from contaminated soil to be inhaled. The model explained two common facts: the failure of cholera always to produce epidemics (conditions were not ripe for the cholera fermentation) and its spontaneous appearance (conditions suddenly became ripe).

But while it held an essential role, the x did not predominate in Pettenkofer's model. It explained some transmission, not causation. Pettenkofer was more interested in the components of y, the factors that would nurture the x and trigger the epidemic. Chief among these were conditions of soil: organic composition, porosity, temperature, moisture. Cholera usually arose, he declared, in a porous x-containing soil, charged with organic matter, and drying out (ground water was falling).

Under such conditions it would take hold in any suitably predisposed population.

Compared to Koch (or Snow), Pettenkofer is obtuse. He appears to be leading researchers into a slough of vaguely defined entities that do not really matter much. Howard-Jones accuses him of violating Occam's razor, the dictum against indiscriminately multiplying explanatory elements. But that view is largely a fossil of the heady simplicity of early bacteriology. Here too it is better to see his views in terms of questions than answers, and to appreciate differing styles of science. Pettenkofer sought the equation of cholera, a model to comprehend the vast and disparate epidemiological data. For the near term, some variables would be underdefined. Most amenable to test were the claims about ground water, but here too the relation was imprecise; anomalies could be explained away by other interfering variables. Koch, on the other hand, would push hard a new analytical tool: ultimately, the culture plate would reveal all, but until then the illuminati must tolerate anomalies and leave some questions hanging. Among these were many of the questions that interested Pettenkofer: why cholera occurred in some places and not others, why at some times and not others, why it disappeared before infecting all, and why it seemed sometimes to spring up without an index case. To followers of Koch, all these could probably be ascribed to a single factor: the presence or absence of the agent, in turn a function of the movement of cholera carriers. In the end, ground water was not so much falsified as forgotten, along with every other geophysical variable. Seed-soil models would re-emerge in the 1930s, though not from the Pettenkoferians.

Our view of Pettenkofer has been retrospective, filtered through the Kochian revolution. At the watershed moment in the early 1880s things looked very different. There was much sound general knowledge of cholera, and a widely held expectation that a microbe agent was involved somehow. As Auguste Hirsch put it: the theory of a living agent "adapts itself to the facts with less constraint than any other, that no fact in the history of cholera goes against it *absolutely*, and that it finds support in many remarkable analogies." Based on the varying circumstances of local outbreaks, Hirsch concluded that the agent was usually inhaled. If it was ingested, food seemed a more prominent vehicle than water. Hirsch was puzzled by the water and cholera controversy: "the opposing views have been put forward in a spirit of extreme one-sidedness." Yet soil and water were not mutually exclusive media, nor need there be only one route into the body. A particulate poison, risen from the soil, might fall on food or get "into wells and other receptacles of water." Future research on the question should "follow a somewhat more rational plan than hitherto." Water analysis was a dead end; so too was the search for "lower organisms." Bettter was to obtain a baseline of the effect of water, which might disclose a transitory choleraic condition. Hirsch cited Snow but without comment.[17]

As well as evaluating rival theories differently from the way we have come to do, some authorities classified them quite differently. One was Henry Bellew, ex-Punjab sanitary commissioner and author of *The History of Cholera in India from 1862 to 1881* (1885).[18] Bellew's main purpose was to reorganize Indian vital and meteorological statistics to make sense of cholera. He did, however, review what he saw as the four prominent theories: "blood-poisoning"; "specific-contagion"; "water contamination by cholera-dejecta"; and "the cholera-germ theory."

"Blood poisoning" reflects the continuing problem of *cholera sicca*, cholera that simply produced sudden collapse. Bellew's contagionism was the classic brand, transmission of a "specific cholera virus" by contact with those "exposed to the influence of the disease" or their clothing or baggage. It no longer seemed plausible to Bellew: cholera did "not travel in all directions as humans do"; it did not occur in proportion to travel. More rapid travel had not increased cholera. Yet in a given location it might arise almost instantaneously. "Water contamination," as we might expect, meant Snow. Bellew saw it as the most popular theory in India (though rejected in England), but as the "least tenable." There was no correlation between any available measures of water quality and cholera. Along the Ganges, cholera moved upstream not down. Bellew conflates Theirsch, Snow, and Koch: a sufferer's dejecta reproduce cholera "only if … swallowed in a certain stage—the vibrio stage—of its decomposition … If the cholera matter have [*sic*] passed this stage it is harmless." Bad water did damage to health and predisposed to cholera.

Bellew's germ theory is one we recognize: "a specific cholera germ or entity endowed with life … which being swallowed in food or water, becomes infinitely multiplied in the intestinal canal, and causes by its action the symptoms which constitute cholera." But it is separate from the contagion and water theories. Worse, he ascribes it to Pettenkofer in one form and in another to the Anglo-Indian J. L. Bryden, who posited a specific cholera wind (the best theory in Bellew's view). Bellew is not mixed up—though often (mis)labeled a miasmatist, Pettenkofer does posit a cholera germ (in 1868 German physicians had found his ideas *too* contagionist). Bellew does, however, reveal the depth of the rational reconstruction that has taken place.[19]

The still special case of India

India would be the test of Snow's ideas, Parkes had claimed. And, if Snow were right, "the prevention of cholera would be easy."[20] And yet, as Bellew pointed out, Anglo-Indian investigators, like their colleagues in Europe, had found that water did not seem to explain cholera. They, like Pettenkofer, sought a cholera equation. A second phase of Indian cholera inquiry began after 1858, following rebellion and transformation of the East India Company's profit fields into Victoria's integrated empire. Newly available statistics finally made it possible to study the temporal and spatial distribution of cholera in a civilian population. Place still mattered, but one does not move a long-standing settlement, or even a village, as one does a regiment. One is facing a phenomenon that appears regularly in some places, and periodically, but seemingly randomly, in others. While in the rest of the world's focus on geographic variables was giving way to interest in contingent factors like the movement of contagious agents or remediable sanitary conditions, in India the trajectory was the opposite. The search for laws of cholera incidence was not obviously or immediately connected to any practical action to prevent the disease. What is inherently geographical may be comprehended but not necessarily prevented.

Positivism persisted in Indian cholera writing. While Bellew will generalize after nearly a thousand pages, he insists on separating the force of fact from gratuitous theory. Theories are partial and contentious. All probably have some merit. We should not expect theoretical agreement; fact is undeniable.

Contemporaries and historians alike have complained that such positivism was itself a theory that served to excuse inaction.

"The idolatry of fact," Sheldon Watts has asserted, was merely British and Anglo-Indian authorities trying to avoid admitting that cholera was contagious and that, in permitting its spread, they were poisoning the world.[21] Positivism and its twin, complexity, brought that great gift of deniability. In a blunt expression of social Darwinism, an American writer declared that

> present knowledge [in 1893] shows that ... [India] is ... responsible [for cholera]. However indifferent we may feel to the annual sacrifice of several hundreds of thousands of natives in India ... [as] application of the theory of the extermination of the unfit and the survival of the fit, we cannot remain indifferent ... when we contemplate the fact that evasions of the responsibility of being our brother's keeper reacts upon ourselves, by perpetuating a disease that may, at any time, invade the countries of the western nations.[22]

Not only were the authorities not taking up their responsibilities as world citizens, they were using the never-ending nature of cholera research as a reason to postpone investing in Indian sanitary infrastructure. (As we shall see, the denial did not stop with Koch's 1883 announcement that he had found the agent of cholera.)

Cholera was indeed a complicated and sensitive issue in Indian politics. Concern to avoid interfering with Hindu fairs or Muslim pilgrimages factored heavily in the government's reluctance to adopt contagionist strategies. The upshot was the promulgation of a doctrine of difference. Cholera was an inherent feature of the timeless east. It is utterly different there. Building on their earlier status as keepers of the facts and therefore true judges of cholera theories, Anglo-Indians countered with their own contemptuous and Conradesque (or Forsterian) narrative. In this, naive Europeans, having magnified coincidence into plausible theory and then announced great truths, sally forth to enlighten India. They must certainly fail, for whoever would really know cholera must know it in India, and those who know it in India know that its depths are unplumbed and perhaps unplumbable. Those who come either leave humbled or go native.

Between the narratives lies an empirical question. How different are the explanatory problems posed by endemic and epidemic disease respectively? Indian cholera was a mix. Where it was endemic, models like Koch's were of little help. India, the Anglo-Indians noted, was far richer in the movement of cholera victims and contamination by cholera excreta than in cases of cholera. Nor did those models seem useful in explaining the periodic, seasonal, and nearly instantaneous eruption of cholera in certain regions, such as coastal east Bengal. Yet endemic cholera was not constant either. Every year did not bring cholera or bring it in the same intensity. Hence, whether it was eternally eastern or not, cholera really was different, at least in parts of India, from the epidemic disease of the rest of the world. Sufficient data might ultimately reveal the laws of its production; to expect also a full understanding of the interplay of multiple mechanisms whose composite action was manifest in those laws was surely overreaching. Learning the laws of cholera might not bring the means to avoid it, but we would not know that until we had learned them.

Koch was no Kurtz. Supremely confident, he would not buy into the myth of India as the graveyard of cholera theories. He would instead, at least for the purposes of cholera science, recolonize India. On his single short visit in 1883–4, Koch blithely bottled and stole the secrets of the exotic orient, if only in print (he did not actually take home a "colony" of the microbe; he

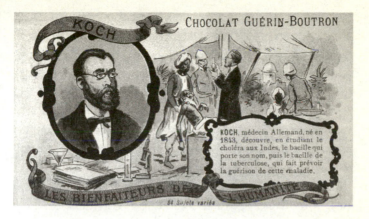

KOCH

CHOCOLAT GUÉRIN-BOUTRON

KOCH, médecin Allemand, né en 1843, découvre, en étudiant le choléra aux Indes, le bacille qui porte son nom, puis le bacille de la tuberculose, qui fait prévoir la guérison de cette maladie.

LES BIENFAITEURS DE L'HUMANITÉ

84 Sujets variés

13. Koch's commanding role in bacteriology admitted even by the French, and celebrated in a chocolate. (*National Library of Medicine*)

soon got a new batch from France, doubtless an equally appropriate collecting site from a Prussian perspective).

Especially when judged in retrospect by those who have arrived at a simple cause with clear-cut prophylactic leverage, other and further research may seem extravagant. In 1884, the equation of cholera with microbe was an audacious act of faith, resting on "extremely shaky foundations," notes Richard Evans.[23] Koch represents the new, Pettenkofer and the Anglo-Indians the old. His victory was also that of laboratory over field, of bacteriology over epidemiology. It represents the emergence of a paradigm that would command the confidence of scientists and society alike in most of the world: all this was clear by the mid 1890s.

But was victory the only possible outcome? And was it really victory? Unabashed, the Anglo-Indians would persist in their cholera heresies, gradually incorporating the cholera microbe into their explanations. Cholera would persist in India after it had receded elsewhere. There was slow progress in prevention and cure after the First World War, yet there cholera was still killing over 200,000 annually (99 per cent of world cholera deaths) at the time of partition and independence. Cholera's etiology turned out to be trickier than Koch had expected. For Koch and for later researchers, India would be the chief field station, a vast laboratory for cholera epidemiology. There the epistemic–ethical conundrum developed in a unique way. Desire to learn about cholera in general often took priority over abatement in particular. It is thus fitting that the research that finally made clear how *Vibrio cholerae* acted was done by two Indian teams in Indian laboratories.

V

CHOLERA GOES INTO
ANALYSIS, AND DIES

"It might be presumed that the contest against epidemics is waged on scientific principles…but unfortunately this is not universally the case; and especially with regard to cholera such a firm basis is wanting." So wrote Robert Koch in 1884.[1] When cholera struck Egypt in 1883, he sought to change that. When he looked down the barrel of his microscope, Koch knew what he was looking for and quickly found it: the comma bacillus, since relabeled (in honor of an earlier observer) *Vibrio cholerae.*

It is hard to miss a watershed in the cholera literature in the 1880s. Tracts and treatises give way to research reports. A cholera of epidemic incidents becomes a cholera of interconnected bacteriological, biochemical, immunological, and pathological problems. Koch's isolation of cholera's agent is a good starting date. Many historical accounts effectively end with it, while a new cholera science starts with it. Epidemiologists may cite Snow; others rarely go back further than Koch.

The post-watershed "scientific" cholera literature reflects and reveres the laboratory, in which the patient seeker, with open-mind and exacting technique, follows an agenda that looks beyond the immediate practical problems of a deadly disease. Surely, progressive knowledge will address human needs, yet one does not expect an end to interesting research problems. One plans lines of experiment in terms of what predecessors and colleagues have done; success is their approbation. Often, experiment led away from the outer world where cholera was experienced and deeper into the controlled world of the laboratory.

Methods had much to do with these changes. The new bacteriology was itself a composite of microscopy and organic chemistry. It would evolve into serology, and would repeatedly be enriched, first by biochemistry, and later by molecular genetics. No less important was the Pearsonian revolution of mathematical techniques for managing variability and helping researchers tease causal inferences from the muddle of disparate fact.

Increasingly, cholera researchers would be professional biomedical scientists. Some would specialize in cholera; for many, cholera-related issues would arise from research programs only incidentally concerned with infectious disease. The prodigious expansion of knowledge, its production through increasingly recondite techniques whose mastery required years of training and the tacit judgment of the expert would transform "cholera" into a composite of specialized knowledge in many fields. By the 1960s, the characteristic form of cholera writing of the nineteenth century—the treatise by a single author who purports to know all relevant facts—had ceased. Pollitzer of the WHO, its last great practitioner in the mid 1950s, took on co-authors for some sections of his great work and was still stretched thin. Comprehensive volumes on cholera would henceforth be compilations. To hope for a God's-eye view of all cholera was to advertise one's naivety, and one's incompetence to achieve that comprehensive perspective with any significant sophistication.

It would be possible to suggest that cholera became a scientific problem as it ceased to be a practical one, but the chronology does not quite work: catastrophic cholera persisted for the first four post-Koch decades, not all of it in places that could be dismissed as irremediably primitive. Initially, the scientific agenda was bound up with practical response, yet the tensions are plain, especially in India, where cholera still ravaged. It too could be a cholera laboratory, one well stocked with experimental subjects. In the 1920s, Felix d'Herelle achieved remarkable results in Indian field trials of a bacteriophage, used as vaccine and as therapeutic agent. His approach was relegated to laboratories, where it languished.[2]

Since 1884, knowledge of cholera has grown greatly, but, as we shall see, the "firm basis" is still wanting. Some quibbled, and still quibble with Koch's assumptions and inferences. The picture has changed remarkably—and repeatedly: if cholera science descends from Koch, it also defies him. Koch equated unique disease with unique organism; twenty-first-century scientists recognize many varieties of *Vibrio cholerae*, gaining or losing pathogenicity as toxin-bearing stretches of DNA move in, or toxin expression is turned up or down in response to environment. They flourish in warm brackish seas as well as human guts, and kill by means that are different from those Koch imagined.

It is better to see Koch as cholera's Lavoisier. His *discoveries* are less important than his transformation of the practice of science—assumptions, techniques, agendas, habits of inference. Most important was an axiom: that the comma bacillus was a distinct entity and the unit of cholera. But Kochian cholera science was much more than *doctrine*. Paradigms, Thomas Kuhn made clear, were traditions of training. Among the sciences, bacteriology stands out as a discipline in which knowledge is guaranteed by mastery of skills learned in the laboratory of a master—like Koch. By the end of 1885 he was already boasting of having taught 150 persons to culture for the comma bacillus.[3] His later career was as institute administrator and host to the legions of foreign researchers who came to learn practical bacteriology. Others went to Paris, though the Pasteurians—wishy-washy on microbe integrity—never had the same clout.

Those who tried to pick up bacteriology from written descriptions of technique in what seemed an easy science (requiring only a modest microscope and a bit of broth) usually found their results written out of the record. Uniformity of method was essential, not only for reliable knowledge but also for intelligible communication. Cooperative endeavor, equally the resolution of controversy, must rest on assumptions of minimal competence. "Much confusion has arisen, owing to differences of opinion among eminent bacteriologists working in different laboratories, as to whether certain strains of comma bacilli were the true organisms of cholera or not," noted the Anglo-Indian pathologist Leonard Rogers in 1911.[4] When Koch referred to "trustworthy observers," he either meant people he had trained or people who got compatible results.[5] In a way that Snow or even Pettenkofer had never done, Koch brought conformity to the science of infectious diseases.

Uniformity of method did not quickly bring clarity. What had seemed simple turned out to be complicated. The central claim that the comma bacillus was the specific agent of cholera would not be generally accepted for about a decade. Even then there was no neat new proof: comma-bacillus-based research had simply achieved an inertial moment that pushed other approaches out of the way. Yet on almost every aspect of cholera science there were conflicting and ambiguous results. For much of the next century, each time researchers felt that the cholera problem had finally been cleared up, anomalies would be discovered, bringing with them recognition of new dimensions of complexity. Mapping these required techniques and instruments that Koch would not recognize, even though they had sometimes descended in a direct line from his work. Often that research was remote from clinical cholera.

Cholera meets Koch

What then did Robert Koch actually do? Cholera occupied only a brief phase of his career. When it broke out in Egypt in 1883, Koch's reputation was peaking: his systematic approach for identifying microbe pathogens had succeeded in the study of anthrax, wound infections, and, most recently, tuberculosis. This incisive bacteriology had come since Europe's last cholera in 1875; there was eagerness to bring it to bear. Hence it was "not unfavourable," as Koch put it, that cholera broke out in Egypt in 1883 (doubtless Egyptians did not see it thus).[6] Discovery of the cholera agent would have a bearing on the vexed question of quarantine, especially in the Suez corridor. It would also be a great catch in the new science. Britain, France, and Germany sent teams to Egypt. The British were interested in sanitary conditions, epidemiology, and defending themselves from the "all-cholera-from-India" charge. The French (Émile Roux, Straus, Thuillier, Nocard) and German commissions (Koch and Georg Gaffky) were fixed on finding the mysterious agent.

The French team returned in September, after Thuillier's death from cholera. Its members thought they had failed. Meanwhile, Koch's team was proposing that a small rod-shaped microbe, present in cholera evacuations in large numbers, might be uniquely associated with cholera. They had seen it in Berlin on slides from Indian victims; they found it in post-mortems in ten Egyptian cholera victims.[7]

Cholera was dying out in Egypt, but Bengal in winter could be trusted for a reliable supply. They arrived in Calcutta in early December. Remarkably, given the antipathy of J. M. Cuningham's Indian medical establishment toward germs, Koch's team was fêted by Cuningham and the government. A genuine intellectual respect to this supercilious German seems unlikely: Koch proposed not only to look for the cholera agent in cadavers, and culture it in animals but also to study its general biology, the effects of disinfectants, the "soil, water, and air in endemic cholera districts," and the relation of cholera to "special characteristics of the population and the environment in endemic cholera areas; outbreaks in prisons, among troops, and on ships; differences between endemic and non-endemic districts; modes of spread of cholera outside endemic districts in and beyond India, and especially the influence of religious customs, pilgrimages, and maritime and land trade routes." In short, he proposed to make quick work of what had occupied, officially or unofficially, a small army of regimental surgeons and district sanitary commissioners for most of a century.[8]

Koch's Calcutta work—December 1883 to April 1884—confirmed and extended his September claim to have identified the agent of cholera. There were three bases of confirmation: first, that the organism was present in all the cholera victims autopsied; second, that it was absent from those who died of other diseases, including diseases of the gut such as diarrhea and dys-entery, and, third, that it could be found in a water tank known to be contaminated with choleraic discharges.[9]

Not until November 1884 could he supplement the Indian evidence with animal experiments and satisfy what are *retrospectively* known as Koch's postulates: a pure culture of an organism associated uniquely with the disease could be introduced into an experimental subject, where it (apparently) produced the disease, then recovered and introduced into a second subject with the same result.[10]

We can assess the claim both in terms of Koch's new rules and in terms of the broader agenda of causal questions outlined earlier. For Koch's genius, like Snow's, lay in simplification, the extraction of questions that could be addressed from the grand mass of fact. The key element of the simplification was to equate all questions of cholera's cause with the doings of the bacillus. In demonstrating that this was the "cause," Koch was helping to change what "cause" meant.

The most comprehensive presentations of Koch's case are in his addresses to the two Berlin conferences on the cholera question in the summer of 1884 and May 1885. In the first of these Koch began by laying out the possible interpretations of a constant relation between a microbe and a disease. The microbe might be cause, consequence, or coincidence. The last seemed intuitively unlikely; the second presumed some unknown element of cholera's pathology that would regularly generate these swarms of unique microbes. That left the third unexcluded possibility, the comma bacillus as cause. In fact, the structure was neither exclusive nor exhaustive, and Koch himself departed from it. The microbe was certainly consequent (the disease process involved production of huge numbers of infective agents); it might be causal as well. Moreover, Koch's tripartite structure suggests that "cause" must be both necessary and sufficient; there is no category for the comma bacillus as one (possibly necessary) component in a more complicated causal process.

Yet in his first address Koch did look at some of these issues in reflecting on how this new discovery might be reconciled with epidemiology and pathology. He acknowledged that mere ingestion of the comma bacillus did not usually bring on cholera. Acidity of the stomach usually killed it; hence he could agree that "predisposition seems to play an important part in cholera-infection. It can be assumed that, of a number of people who are exposed to cholera-infection, only a fraction of them fall ill, and that these are almost always those already suffering from some kind of digestive disturbance." That "disturbance" might be a catarrh or simply overeating (large, underdigested boluses of food would protect the bacteria until they had passed into the more congenial environment of the small intestine). Koch was reckoning here with the infrequency of communication of the disease—a well-founded fact of cholera, long at the heart of anticontagionist arguments. He was also accommodating the frequent association of cholera with general ill health and poverty, and with the roles of premonitory diarrhea, unease, and even, perhaps, anxiety.

Equally, he enlisted the perspectives of the sanitarians and so-called localists in speculating about means of transmission: the bacillus was probably transmitted by dirty hands, possibly by flies. Most often it was transmitted by water, particularly water that had percolated through ground saturated with organic matter. He had found that the microbe did not do well in spring or river water; it needed a richer organic medium.

We can, then, very easily demonstrate the connection between the ground water and the spread of cholera. Everywhere…water stagnates on the surface, or in the ground, in marshes, in docks which have no outlet, in places where the ground is formed like a trough, in sluggish rivers, and the like, the conditions which have been described can be found. There a concentrated nutrient solution can form in the neighborhood of animal and vegetable decaying matters most easily, and give the micro-organisms opportunity for growth.

Koch goes on, sounding ever more Pettenkoferian: "the connection between the sinking of the ground water and the increase of many infective diseases we might explain thus: That with the sinking of the ground water the current which exists in it becomes very much lessened." There will be less water, thus more concentrated nutriment. And he clarifies his position on the contested question of cholera as a waterborne disease:

> Though I have cited…examples of the advantages of a good supply of drinking water, the assurance that I am not a supporter of the exclusive drinking-water theory is scarcely necessary…I want specially to avoid any prominent point of view, for I consider that the ways in which cholera can spread itself are extremely different, and that almost every place has its own peculiarities…Regulations…for the prevention of infection….must be drawn up, accordingly.[11]

During that first year a good deal of work was done in Koch's laboratory and others to get a fix on the natural history of the comma bacillus. Many studied its survival in water. Koch himself certainly thought it could flourish outside the human body, in any warm, wet, and nutrient-rich environment.

Here Koch sounds like Acland or Pettenkofer. Are we seeing here a junior deferring to a senior colleague? Koch needed allies.

He was indeed in a weaker position than a year later once he had coerced the comma bacillus into multiplying in the guts of guinea pigs. And yet we would be wrong to ascribe too much to a rift with Pettenkofer that would be severe a few years hence.

Much ado about laundry

Precisely because the rift would become so bitter and has been seen as fundamental, it is useful to recognize how narrow was the conceptual gap between Kochians and Pettenkoferians. Divergence was never inevitable; it reflected priorities, institutions, and egos. The gravest problem both faced was not why there was cholera, but why there was not more cholera. Koch, and Snow before him, had held that filth was not enough; you needed specific germs. Pettenkofer held that germs were not enough; you needed some special filth as medium. But Koch appealed to media too. The reason that ingestion of the comma bacillus only rarely produced cholera was that the internal environment was only rarely suitable.

During the mid 1880s both sides struggled to make sense of the role of contaminated linens in cholera transmission. The European outbreak of 1884 had been attributed to the return to France of the clothing of a colonial soldier, who had died of cholera in South East Asia.

It is common to see such transmission by fomites as a special case of contagion. Yet, when Hirsch discussed the frequent appearance of cholera following the arrival of "linen, bedding, or clothes, soiled by the dejecta of cholera patients," he saw this, not as contagion, but in Pettenkoferian "seed and soil" terms: the dirty linen ignited combustible conditions, setting off cholera.[12] Koch's most important British critic, Edward Klein, offered the analogy of food poisoning. Food (a medium) plus a microbe yielded a toxin known as a ptomaine. If a combination of factors was required, it was moot which was seed and which was soil. The linens could be either: perhaps they conveyed the igniter or perhaps the dried evacuations were the crucial medium that some widely distributed microbe required to produce the cholera ferment. The arrival of the missing ingredient explained the occasional explosiveness of cholera—zero to epidemic within half an hour. That explosiveness seemed incompatible with the person-to-person spread of classic contagionism.[13]

Koch, who wished to see linens merely as vehicles for microbe transport, faced the problem that cholera-causing linens were often dry and had traveled long and far. The comma bacillus, on the other hand, was short-lived and required a warm and wet medium. In vain, Koch sought for a resting or spore stage that would resolve this anomaly. No matter: transmission of cholera in contaminated linens would simply become a mode of contagion and vindication of Koch. Whether or not the comma bacillus should survive the trip, it evidently did. Co-factors were moot; cholera's explosiveness might be explained by mass contamination of food or water. So well did Koch succeed that it has been hard to see how linens might have been interpreted differently.

Boss Koch

Koch's address to the second Berlin conference on the cholera question in May 1885 reflects a change in tone. He was no longer interested in indulging Pettenkoferian crotchets. By that time Koch felt that he had demonstrated that the microbe was not merely a consequence, but cause. He had—he thought—produced cholera in an animal model. In early summer 1884 Koch had learned that the physiologists Nicati and Reitsch had induced the comma bacillus to kill guinea pigs. They had ligated the bile duct and injected the bacillus directly into the small intestine, but the effect (in Koch's view) was hardly analogous to natural cholera and might be an artifact of the operation. Koch tried oral administration, neutralizing the stomach acid to allow the bacillus to pass intact into the small intestine, but this failed until he supplemented it with injection of opium into the small intestine to slow peristalsis. Thus administered, the microbe killed the animal, could be recovered in pure culture, and then cause disease in another. Koch had also chanced on an obscure report by Macnamara. An Indian water tank, much like that from which he had cultured the comma bacillus, had received a known contamination of cholera excreta; fifteen persons promptly came down with the disease.

These fueled his confidence, but Koch was also on the defensive, for there were now critics. This first generation of critics held either that comma bacilli were common (therefore presumably innocent) or that other organisms were guilty of causing cholera-like diseases. One, the Finkler–Prior bacillus, which had similar characteristics in culture to Koch's organism, was presented as the cause of *cholera nostras*.

Koch was generally uninterested and unrepentant. His defiance did much to shape subsequent cholera research. A tentative stance—there is an apparent link between cholera and a comma-shaped bacillus, but it is not clear how distinct this organism is or why it only sometimes causes cholera—was rejected for a doctrinaire one: the comma bacillus was a species whose presence was congruent with that of true cholera and whose discovery pre-empted all other questions.

For the next several decades, the distribution of clinical cholera would be treated more in terms of the distribution of the agent than of that agent's interactions with environment or host. That agent did not merely contribute to a complicated cholera process; it, and it alone, caused a distinct disease. The determinative bacteriology of what we now know as *Vibrio cholerae* would become the central problem of cholera research: by what combination of characteristics in growth media could the particular toxic microbe that always causes cholera be distinguished from its many imposters? Even the mechanism of its toxicity would be secondary.

The change is evident in the gradual exclusion of predisposition. In 1884 Koch had accepted that "predisposition seems to play an important part in cholera infection." Any remote factor that disturbed the gut might aid the cholera bacillus. A year later the power of the agent was predominant: "the cholera bacteria have extremely energetic pathogenic properties, and are able to show them, if they reach the small intestine uninjured, and find it in a condition which allows them to obtain a firm footing and to develop." The complexity of predisposition had been reduced to stomach acidity.[14] As the stomach was now deemed acid-free *except* when there was food to digest, there were no exogenous factors to block its lethal work. Nothing here was incompatible with the earlier treatment, but the emphasis had shifted: as the microbe loomed larger all else receded.

Koch was also hinting that all the many geographic factors posited to account for the uneven spread of cholera could be reduced to varying degrees of population immunity. He estimated that a case of cholera left one immune for three or four years (modern authorities would agree). Hence the reason cholera moved only northwest from the pilgrimage sites at Hardwar was because there was high endemicity in other directions; in effect, they led to burnt-over territory. No longer was there need to kowtow about ground water; rather, Koch accused Pettenkofer of intentionally ignoring induced immunity. Koch noted also the higher attack rate among European than among native Indian soldiers and the Indian government's policy of using Indian nurses on cholera cases.

Equally ad hoc, at least for the time being, with the immunity explanation for the absence of cholera was the explanation of (apparently) spontaneous outbreaks by appeal to asymptomatic carriers or unrecognized mild cases. In July 1884 Koch had faced the problem directly. "I could only answer, that the mode of introduction...had not yet been made clear; but...the origin of the cholera...must be traced back to India." He had admitted that he could not prove a negative: that cholera was never spontaneous was a matter of "conviction." But only assume that cholera was imported and it would be opponents who bore the burden of proving the negative: they could never claim that there *had not* been some hidden contact; cholera's presence was proof that there had been. But here, too, the hypotheses of temporary immunity and asymptomatic carriers did not logically exclude the environmental and social factors that had been so prominent in earlier cholera epidemiology.[15]

Koch's reductionist reading of cholera was largely in place by mid 1885. Given equal means for fecal–oral transmission within a locality, cholera's presence was a function of the presence of its carriers, symptomatic or not; its absence was a function of their absence or of the presence of a high level of immunity. The emphasis on the presence or absence of the agent as the sole independent variable has been defended as appropriate application of the principle of parsimony. If all plausibly follows from these, why posit further factors?

But Koch's adoption of these positions was less a matter of adherence to Occamite principles than an effort to shake off critics by resetting the agenda of cholera research. Matters had become polarized. Pettenkofer was not amenable to sharing power with a younger rival; though finally persuaded, the Pasteur-led French had taken umbrage at Koch's audacity in studying the French epidemic in the summer of 1884. In India, where so many had spent years on the cholera puzzle, it rankled that an upstart German should solve it in a few, relatively leisurely months; while the British worried that the comma bacillus would invite Suez quarantines (though Koch, like many other neo-contagionists, doubted the effectiveness of such approaches).

Cholera finds an advocate

The most trenchant of the early critics was the Austro-English physiologist-bacteriologist Edward Emanuel Klein, head of the Brown Animal Sanatory Institute in London. A disciple neither of Pasteur nor of Koch, Klein has been marginalized in a heritage that celebrates discovery over skeptical critique. With a junior colleague, Henneage Gibbes, Klein had been sent by the British government to India in the summer of 1884 to test Koch's claims. (Klein was the senior colleague; his *The Bacteria of Asiatic of Cholera* (1886) includes large passages from the report.) On the basis of their report (though, evidently, without Klein's active involvement), the British government would issue an "official refutation" of Koch.[16] Enlisted to defend the statistical approach of the Anglo-Indian sanitarians, Klein, even more than Koch, pushed cholera into the laboratory.

What Klein offered was a critique equally of method and of inference. Initially, he did not say that Koch had been wrong and some other theory was right; he simply accused Koch of going beyond what the evidence would allow. But, even as their disagreement sharpened, Klein continued to play an ambiguous role. Sometimes he confirmed Koch; often he did not; he was neither friendly critic nor obdurate opponent. Koch, however, saw Klein as out to get him: "he has exclusively busied himself in upsetting my statements."[17]

Klein (and Gibbes) offered three critiques—one based in pathology, a second in microscopy, and a third epidemiological.

Klein could not replicate all of Koch's results in animal experiments. Hence he concluded that Koch's guinea pigs had not been killed by cholera; rather their deaths had been an artifact of experiment. He placed Koch's results in a long line of experiments in which presumptive cholera agents had been administered by various routes to various animal subjects, whose succumbing was invariably interpreted as cholera. One might include Orton's lowered air pressure; also the administration of hydrogen sulfide or cholera blood. Often the animals died. Hardly surprising, noted Hirsch, who had addressed the issue earlier: "The experiment-animals were subjected to unusual conditions of living; they were not rarely exposed to tortures; blood serum and bowel-discharges were poured through them by the ounce." Often the stomach or bowels were affected, but the pathology was not unambiguously cholera. Yet negative results—the apparent failure of hypothesized agents to produce cholera—meant nothing either; it remained "unsettled whether those classes of the animal kingdom…possess any susceptibility to the cholera poison at all."[18]

Koch had recognized the problem. In moving away from the Nicati–Rietcsh approach in which a culture was implanted surgically, and toward oral administration, he was trying to avoid the complication that the guinea pigs might be dying from the operation not the agent. Some of his experiments were controlled, and Koch was confident that he could prevent surgical septicemia. Yet Klein objected even to the injection of opium; he found that the mode of injecting opium significantly affected the outcome. He objected also that Koch's guinea pigs had no cholera symptoms: they suffered from a "paralytic weakness of the hinder extremities, coldness of the head and legs, and prolonged [slowed] respiration." They did not have diarrhea. Moreover, guinea pigs that had received doses of other microbes by the same route also died.[19]

Klein saw nothing that would rule out the view of the comma bacillus as a "consequence": that it flourished in the guts of guinea pigs in conjunction with fatal pathological effect did not prove that the flourishing caused the effect. If one assumed, as Klein did, that the technique of introducing the bacillus itself damaged the animal, that conclusion was the more unlikely. He saw Koch's microbe as an opportunistic saprophyte that preyed on tissue already destroyed, whether by the true cause of cholera or by the surgical interventions of the operator. It also produced a ptomaine that killed the animals. Recovery of the microbe and reintroduction into a new animal was no more conclusive: it simply repeated the error. And what of negative experiments? Koch and others had frequently failed to produce cholera in their test animals. If the introduction of the microbe did not always produce this "cholera" (which had no cholera symptoms), one might conclude that one was looking not at the cholera microbe at all, but at some generic infection.[20]

If not the comma bacillus, what then caused cholera? Klein and Gibbes held that Koch was looking too far down the intestine, where post-mortem damage was likely. Further up, they found a characteristic coccus in mucus lumps. This seemed a likelier candidate as a cholera cause. It was in cholera vomit, too. Yet they did not propose it as the cholera agent. More important was to show how readily wishful thinking might be indulged in bacteriology. Koch was guilty of guilt by association.

One should also look at an earlier stage. Koch boasted of rapid autopsy. But if the comma bacillus were consequent rather than cause, thriving in the detritus of the cholera-damaged gut, the rapidity of autopsy should make a major difference. Autopsy fifteen minutes or a half hour after death should reveal fewer of the comma bacillus than Koch's typical three or four hours. But Klein's own results were inconclusive.

Finally, they appealed to the old chestnut of anticontagion. If cholera were contagious, more people—the medical staff of cholera hospitals or residents living near the tank from which Koch had isolated the comma bacillus—should be getting it. (If stomach acid was the impeding factor, it would impede too much.) Revisiting the same tank from which Koch had isolated the comma bacillus, they found it full of such organisms. Yet, "notwithstanding their presence in this water, and...the extensive use the 200 families were constantly making of it, there has been no outbreak of cholera." Here, in the terms of Snow, was "an experiment performed by nature on a scale large enough to serve as an absolute and exact one." If there were so much cholera in India, there must be much contagion. If it were communicated by filth, particularly filthy water, there was a superfluity. Koch had certainly shown that enormous quantities of comma bacilli were excreted; in India they "find constantly and copiously access" to human bodies.[21] With so many comma bacilli, where was the missing cholera?

Klein and Gibbes also objected that Koch had stripped down expectations of explanation in failing to explain *how* the comma bacillus was supposed to be causing cholera. Koch, like Pettenkofer, had posited a toxin. To Pettenkofer, the production of the cholera ptomaine by some peculiar fermentation of soil organic matter was a working hypothesis. Ultimately, it might explain isolated outbreaks where no prior contact with cholera existed—a domain that Koch summarily denied. Pettenkofer was appealing to a Newtonian model of explanation: a unique set of conditions must exist to generate this poison, but, once generated, it must cause cholera.

For Koch, all those unique conditions were presumably embodied in the comma bacillus. He too had assumed (rightly) that the comma bacillus wreaked its havoc by means of a ptomaine-like toxin, and (wrongly) that the toxin operated systemically (that is, throughout the body, probably by means of the blood). Having failed to find the organism in the blood, he had ceased to worry overmuch about how it did what it did: the specificity of the microbe was to be sufficient explanation for the specificity of the pathological process. As van Heyningen and Seal would observe a century later, Koch's ptomaine assumption was gratuitous: "a notion that easily sprang to mind and filled the vacuum that existed for want of any other explanation for the harmful effects of infectious diseases."[22]

There is no little irony here: one proposes a cause for cholera, a pathological process, which fails even to produce a characteristic pathology or to produce it invariably. In practice, the finding of cause deflected the need to explain. Throughout the long history of cholera, the pathology of the disease had been equally as interesting as its causation, and the two inquiries had been linked: to understand what was happening within the stricken body seemed likely to illuminate how that condition had come about. As William Coleman has pointed out, one reason the French Cholera Commission did not immediately grasp the importance of the comma bacillus was that it had broader expectations of what criteria a proposed cholera cause must satisfy. On the principle that the cause must act through the blood, they looked there. (So too, initially, did Koch.) They assumed also that effect should be proportionate to cause: one should find the greatest quantity of causal agent in the most rapid and intense cholera. That was *cholera sicca*, which did not involve diarrhea and did not produce large quantities of comma bacillus. Koch, on the other hand, treated both the failure to find bacteria in the blood and the ever-vexing problem of *cholera sicca*, along with the larger inability to say anything definitive about pathology, as matters that could be bypassed for the present. (Klein did demonstrate a lack of relation between intensity of cholera and number of comma bacilli.)

For Klein and Gibbes, the upshot was that the comma bacillus was not the cause of cholera, though it was a typical product and might therefore have diagnostic significance.

Doubting is easy. Always, some bloody-minded skeptic can be found to gainsay whatever seminal transformation is in the works. Hence Klein has been seen as conducting a futile (even disingenuous) rearguard action against the germ-theory juggernaught. He cannot conclusively refute; by creating just enough doubt, he produces the goods Britain needs: deniability remains plausible a while longer; pressure to quarantine Suez shipping can be deflected on the contrived uncertainty of junk science.

But such a reconstruction requires enlistment of a bacteriological paradigm that had yet fully to triumph. Klein and Gibbes were tough critics. They did not extend Koch any benefit of doubt. Sometimes Klein discounts Koch's efforts to deal with precisely the problems he has raised. Yet, if one starts with Klein's saprophyte hypothesis, most phenomena of the comma bacillus are plausibly explained. And Koch's rejoinders were equally tendentious. He had published his cholera claim at an audaciously early stage of investigation and doggedly defended both its accuracy as an empirical finding and its adequacy as a causal explanation. He resisted complexity, and steered inquiry away from other vibrios that caused diarrhea (classed as "non-cholera vibrios" or NCVs, these would be neglected for decades), as well as from comma vibrios that apparently did not cause cholera (long known collectively as non-O1). In the emerging paradigm, commonalities among vibrios and generalizations about their natural history would be much less important than seeking to define the unique properties of the particular entity that generated cholera.

Often, later research would reiterate these early criticisms. The assumption that any toxic effect of the cholera bacillus was cholera would turn out to be unfounded; the microbe carried more than one toxin. Koch's legatees would become comfortable with the admission that only some comma bacilli (those possessing the so-called cholera toxin) cause cholera and do so only under some conditions. Yet these would be refinements not refutations.

Koch was extraordinarily successful as a paradigm-builder (indeed one is tempted to see him as the paradigmatic paradigm builder). But ways of seeing are equally ways of not seeing. Klein and Gibbes, like Pettenkofer, sought a theory "capable

of explaining all the facts concerning cholera."[23] In that macroscopic perspective some variables were necessarily defined
empirically, i.e., only in terms of their effects. Koch, on the other
hand, had a fine sense of Medawar's "art of the soluble." He had
developed powerful methods that could drive a research program. Given the irresolution of the previous half century, there
was good reason to focus, even at the cost of oversimplifying.

And, yet, the movement into the laboratory was to create an
ever greater distance between cutting-edge research and clinical and epidemiological cholera. This persisted for decades,
notwithstanding periodic admissions that truths of the laboratory were not borne out in the field. Even in the laboratory, what
would be seen as fruitful lines of research were not always fully
followed up—such as the observation of Nicati and Reitsch that
a cell-free filtrate of the cholera bacillus *also* killed guinea pigs
with symptoms of septic infection, in retrospect an opening to
explore the operation of cholera's toxin(s).

The full range of issues did not go away. When, in the 1990s,
cholera science would finally break free (making the laboratory
adjunct rather than prison), the new cadre of researchers would
sometimes wonder why there had been so little work on what
seemed obvious questions. They had simply not gone back far
enough. It would also be complained that a great deal of twentieth-century cholera research was simply irrelevant—able work,
perhaps, but tied to erroneous assumptions.

Hamburg

The outbreak of cholera at Hamburg in the autumn of 1892
(and at nearby Altona in January 1893) has generally been seen
as proof positive: whatever the skeptics might say, Koch had

indeed found the right bug. It is also often seen an exemplar of faith in the direct applicability of science to cholera control. Had the world only listened to Koch, or earlier to John Snow, all would have been well. But, instead, many had listened to the well-meaning if egocentric Pettenkofer, whose ineffabilities were often seized upon as a means to deflect needed change into cynical or self-interested symbolic sanitarianism. The result was confusion, delay, even subversion. In Naples this meant airy avenues and wholesale slum cleansing rather than better water; in Hamburg, a ready apologetic for a dangerous water supply.

The Hamburg epidemic did alter the balance of probability. Koch did win; Pettenkofer really did lose. But the contest was less decisive than many think it should have been. Older and other explanations remained logically possible; the cholera in Hamburg and Altona was more complicated in epidemiology and ambiguous in implications than many accounts recognize.

The epidemic shared important features with Snow's seminal cases: adjacent places different in water supply had quite different experiences with cholera. Hanseatic Hamburg, long run by a merchant oligopoly fixated on profit at the expense of public works, would confirm the Ackerknechtian antinomies: commercial domination was coupled with anticontagionism. Hamburg would come to epitomize sanitarian false consciousness. There, as in the British-held Suez, was gold in plausible deniability. The refugees from the shtetls might be dirty and disgusting, but they constituted no epidemic threat and could be moved quickly on to America. When epidemics came, Hamburg's leaders maundered on about bad airs and made minimal efforts to clean the streets and feed the poor, but they would not invest in the expert-based infrastructure that might really make a difference: a safe and plentiful water supply. The epidemic of August to November 1892, fatal in about half of the 16,000 cases, was largely restricted to Hamburg. That great port relied primarily on water from upstream on the Elbe. Downstream Altona, a working-class suburb, had taken steps to protect water quality. Its raw water came from a worse source than Hamburg's, the tidal Elbe, but the water was filtered, and the filtered water was checked weekly for coliform bacteria by well-trained technicians.

The theory of the "revered Herr Localist" (Pettenkofer) could not be right, Koch would write; by his theory, cholera should have struck both places symmetrically. By 1893 the balance of power between Koch and Pettenkofer had shifted; as the sarcasm suggests, Koch, imperial and imperious in Berlin, no longer had need to suffer Pettenkofer.[24]

Yet, when cholera returned in January 1893, it was largely exclusive to Altona, clearly transmitted by the filtered water supply that Koch had so lavishly praised. Quite as much as Hamburg's, Altona's experience confirmed cholera as waterborne. It did reveal, however, the broad gulf between science and effective technical response. The Altona outbreak was the second occasion of a filtered water supply causing an urban cholera outbreak: for many, the east London cholera of 1866 had been the convincing proof of transmission by (filtered) water. Koch could pin down the time of the breakdown in filtration, he could say which filter had failed, but he could not prevent breakdowns. A network for distributing safe water could spread deadly cholera equally well.

To Koch, the simple lesson of Hamburg had been: "invest in sound waterworks; your penny-wise pound-foolish public health policies will only bring on more cholera." And yet, as with quarantines, more precise knowledge of the microbial agent of disease transmission might offer unambiguous sanction for a technical goal, while at the same time rendering its achievement problematic. Usually in the modern Western world the answer to problems like "how can one guarantee Altona's filters?" has been "spend more on research." There are other answers: to change institutions of administration, or to transform through some defensible public process the public willingness to incur risks in some areas to gain benefits in others. But the "more-research" answer seems to bypass a need for tradeoffs; it is a solution to messy and unresolvable conflict within communities where power is usually unequally distributed in the first place. More research on the viability of the comma bacillus in relation to the construction and management of water filters may show that what appear zero-sum games are not, and there are usually capable researchers willing to do the work. Sometimes it works, sometimes not.

In the case of cholera, this hope proved over-optimistic. As Koch himself had recognized and as modern experts reiterate, there are many occasions for fecal–oral transmission—by food, by in-home water storage, by lack of adequate handwashing, and so forth. Damning one mode of transmission may not increase the pressure on others, but it does nothing to relieve that pressure either. And cholera was a far more variable and adaptable entity than Koch, shrewd as he was, could appreciate in the 1890s. Many sensed that complexity; Pettenkoferian views did not quickly disappear after 1892. And, where money to improve water works was the limiting factor, more science might have been to no avail.

The lesson of Hamburg was important. It did not inspire a revolution in water supply, for one was well under way, pushed along by industrial water needs, by universal water-closeting and other bourgeois hygienic expectations, and even by a general recognition of the possibility of eliminating waterborne diseases, rather than as a specific strategy of cholera prevention. In any case, cholera was disappearing from the north and the west. More than ever, cholera would be "Asiatic." It would fester on, but in India, or inner Asia, or even perhaps Russia or China, vast places with lives to spare. Much of the cholera in those places was in villages, where people took water from wells, ponds, or rivers. Often safe mains water was out of the question, dismissed on grounds of cost or of race: the health of native populations was not really remediable and hence did not really matter. What could be done, like the boiling of water, had to be done by the people themselves. If villagers with their barbaric customs chose not to take these steps, well, that was that.

Needles and fluids

Yet primarily it was not quarantines, nor India, nor even the empirical success of Hamburg that transformed cholera science, but the laboratory itself. Whatever its ultimate relation to cholera might prove to be, the comma bacillus represented something novel in the history of cholera: an *apparently* unambiguous entity that could be the subject of experiment. *In fact*, it turned out be an ambiguous entity, vastly more complicated and variable than was appreciated in the late 1880s.

Prior to staining and culturing techniques, which transformed the bacillus from curiosity of natural history to analytical instrument, the only experimental systems for cholera had been analytical chemistry and pathophysiology. Not only did the chemists fail to find anything unique in choleraic water or air, sometimes, as in the case of water from the Broad Street pump, their findings were the opposite of what epidemiology would have led them to expect: Broad Street water was purer by their measures than waters not linked to cholera. In physiology, methodological anarchy prevailed: plenty of experimentation, little uniformity, scant rigor, wildly divergent conclusions. Statistics, too, may qualify as an experimental system, yet the lack of a standard diagnosis of cholera, the lack of any systematic attempt to measure cases as well as deaths, and, in many places, the abysmal quality of record-creating institutions undercut confidence in comparative studies; even had the data been better, the mathematics had yet to be developed.

In contrast, the experimental system of more-or-less standardized culture media, more-or-less standardized experimental animals, and the ability to control physical and chemical parameters of time, temperature, pH, and so forth had great promise as means for producing knowledge that was replicable if not necessarily relevant. Before 1884 virtually anyone could enter the lists of cholera research; by 1885 Koch was reading confirmations of his findings (or failures to confirm) in terms of adequate instruments. Adequate training would soon be even more important. Henceforth, to contribute, one pretty well had to have, even if indirectly, the imprimatur of Koch or Pasteur (or even, for a while, Pettenkofer, whose students were well dug in and would assimilate the Kochian revolution on their own terms). An insular British bacteriology would struggle. Despite the support of Lord Lister, William Watson Cheyne, pupil of Koch and Klein's nemesis, was never able to establish hegemony over the motley collection of physiologists and chemists who dabbled with greater or lesser competence and confidence.

The laboratory was the home of cholera for most of the twentieth century. Its prominence would lead to a split in what "cholera" signified. In some parts of the world the locking of cholera into the laboratory coincided with its disappearance: no longer did people die of cholera, no longer did the prospect of cholera warrant investment of anxiety. Elsewhere, where cholera still prevailed, people often found themselves locked in a laboratory with it, a laboratory with boundaries but not walls. To be part of a grand epidemiological experiment was not necessarily a bad thing, yet the priorities of the laboratory generally dominated. Uniformity, replicability, and accountability might trump applicability and bypass relevance. The laboratory setting could nurture strains of cholera inquiry, allowing promising insights to survive beyond initial failures. Yet the flip side was acceptance of laboratory-defined norms, with regard not only to empirical success, but to research priorities, the scope for individual initiative, and operant codes of ethics. Almost always the moral tales from this age of laboratory cholera are double-edged.

The tale of Jaime (or Jaume) Ferrán's cholera vaccine is one of tragedy. Cholera hit Spain hard in 1884, continuing into 1885. The epidemic came presumably from France, via Algeria. During 1884 Ferrán, a general practitioner from Tortosa, had been sent by the Barcelona authorities to observe cholera at Marseilles and Toulon. During these months he decided to see if what was true for smallpox was true for cholera. Would inducing a weak cholera prevent one from getting a strong cholera? That led first to experiments on guinea pigs, then to self-inoculation, and on to trials on Barcelonan physician-comrades in March 1885. On May 1 Ferrán began intramuscular injections of a pure culture of the comma bacillus on volunteers in Alcira. In all, about 30,000 would be inoculated. The results appeared impressive. Roughly a third were done in the city of Valencia. There, about 9 percent of the un-inoculated population were attacked by cholera, compared to 2 percent of those who had received one injection, and 0.72 percent of those who had received two. Inoculees who got cholera were said to have milder and shorter cases. Yet the Spanish authorities were unenthusiastic. Ostensibly their concern was that the reaction at the injection site was not mild cholera but a general infection that might become septicemia. Some saw Ferrán as a charlatan, using Koch's reputation to sell bogus inoculations to desperate people.

If the Spanish authorities were merely irritated by this maverick who seemed cavalier with the lives of his countrymen, others had more to lose. Ferrán was that most dangerous of species, an independent bacteriologist. A steady series of remarkable claims came from his household lab. Others had great difficulty infecting guinea pigs with cholera; not so Ferrán. Koch had searched for a resting (spore) stage of the comma bacillus; Ferrán claimed to have found one. At stake was the credibility of institutionalized bacteriology, not merely the replicability of particular claims. Particularly uneasy were the French, for Pasteur was master of all vaccines. All Europe investigated him, Ferrán complained: seventeen scientific academies, twelve medical societies, seven institutes, eight medical faculties. Pasteur himself was open-minded and Chauveau encouraging, but most could not stomach the idea of an unknown local doctor in a backward nation overthrowing serious science. Their responses ranged from outright repudiation—Ferrán must be wrong—to dismissal: nothing could be known, for this was Spain and the vital statistics were all lies.

The American reporter Shakespeare offered a sympathetic, if calculated, endorsement, however: Ferrán's comma-bacillus-based vaccine confirmed Koch; Koch was the route to better border security. Induced immunity would grease the skids of commerce and colonialism; vaccination would save the lives of the slovenly masses who would never willingly be clean, but would get a shot; in times of panic "such a harmless and ... apparently uninjurious means ... would be most willingly and widely submitted to) ..."[25]

Having been kitted out in Berlin with the junior bacteriologist's kit, Shakespeare arrived in Spain with low expectations. He had been repeatedly warned off—no serious scientist would come close to Ferrán. But how to judge? Remarkably, Shakespeare, like the august French team that had visited a year earlier, was less interested in the results themselves than the likelihood that Ferrán *could* produce good results; was he in fact a hitherto unrecognized member of the League of Bacteriological Gentlemen. Like the French, Shakespeare was not at first impressed. One room of Ferrán's "modest" home was a laboratory. There was none of the "scrupulous cleanliness" of the bacteriological laboratory (and there was no obvious water closet), but one of the two microscopes was a new Hartnack. He decided that good work could be done in such a setting. The French commissioners—Brouardel, Charrin, and Albarran—had made the setting equally central in deciding that good work could not be done. There were no facilities for experimental animals (Ferrán claimed to have finished with animal work) or staining materials. The media appeared sterile, but the incubator lacked a means of temperature regulation. They reported two microscopes, but not the Hartnack.

The French relied on impressions, because they and Ferrán had quickly arrived at an impasse. The commissioners were not colleagues coming to learn, as Ferrán had hoped; they came either to expose fraud or to steal his discovery. He complained of their "marked air of superiority" and "mortifying suspiciousness." Hence he offered them proof, but not credibility—he would make their culture into a vaccine, but he would not let them watch. This was not satisfactory: results did not speak for themselves; confidence came from skill and technique. Making virus into vaccine by attenuation was hard even for Pasteur. Without exacting protocols, uniformity would be impossible; without transparency of procedure, there could be no ethical warrant for use of Ferrán's vaccine. Sooner or later, he would have to go public; he could not vaccinate all. And if the vaccine worked as well as he claimed, every day of secrecy was morally irresponsible.

While Ferrán's concerns about credit are plausible and his humiliation understandable, it is likely that a main reason for keeping the attenuation procedure secret was that there was not one. Ferrán claimed to know how to attenuate but found it unnecessary. He injected pure culture. The dose, combined with injection into the arm, a tissue remote from the central site of choleraic activity, together produced the necessary mitigating effect. This was no secret; the commissioners, however, were evidently thinking exclusively in terms of vaccine development as it took place in the Pasteurian universe.

Shakespeare was more flexible. Ferrán did not demonstrate processes—it is not clear that Shakespeare asked him to—but he did demonstrate technical skills—taking a tiny drop of culture by sterilized rod into a new gelatine tube, staining and mounting slides. Shakespeare was impressed: "beautifully stained" slides on a par with the best work; "indicative of *habitual* practice of no mean skill." Having discovered what Ferrán could do, Shakespeare moved on to what he knew, and found him sound on theory and practice. Ferrán passed: a "quiet, reserved, courteous, intelligent, and generally well informed physician."[26]

Ferrán's attitude was that he was merely saving lives—all anyone should care about. An investigation by the Spanish Academy of Medicine set out the issues clearly. Generally the commissioners were cautious, recommending animal tests and trials on small populations (Ferrán had done both). A minority objected to the freedom of any practitioner to expose a population to an unproven agent. While acknowledging margin of safety issues, the majority held it unlawful to restrain medical practice. Individual doctors, not the state, bore responsibility for care.

Shakespeare agreed: practicing medicine always and necessarily involved experimenting on human beings. Certainly he was correctly representing the legacy of cholera therapy. In a disease so deadly, plausibility had always been warrant enough. He did not see artificial induction of disease into persons not yet exposed as significantly different. In fact, though there were mutterings that Ferrán's vaccine harmed or even killed, the paragons of Pasteurian science were less concerned with safety or effectiveness than with replicability. Knowing what was going into Spanish arms was more important than knowing whether it worked. The Belgian commission, Ferrán complained, wanted only to know how he had managed to kill guinea pigs when others found this so difficult.

Within the decade, cholera inoculation would be taken up in India by one with proper Pasteurian credentials, Waldemar Haffkine. For decades, Haffkine struggled for uniformity in his cultures. He developed an elaborate strategy to enhance virulence (and thereby to strengthen sera) by passing the culture through guinea pigs and other animals. In colonial India, he had access to groups of experimental subjects—the military, or

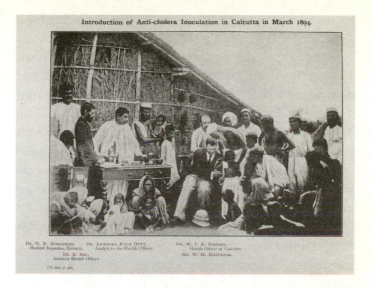

14. Cholera vaccination in India. (*Wellcome Library, London*)

workers on tea plantations—who were seemingly more tractable than the motley crowd Ferrán had vaccinated in liberalizing
Spain. To Haffkine, the amateur Ferrán was not even a precur-
sor who had been superseded, but a dangerous quack.

Yet Haffkine's results were usually not markedly superior
to Ferrán's. One may sympathize with both sides. The French
commissioners cringed (as we do too) when Ferrán inoculated
twenty nuns with the same needle, unsterilized, and seemed
oblivious to air bubbles in his syringe. Yet he vaccinated as
a medical practitioner, on willing, yet desperate persons for
whom an imperfect vaccine was a good bet in the face of a
deadly disease. Haffkine operated as a scientist injecting subjects on terms not set by the injectees. Ironically, later vaccine
researchers would complain that Haffkine's promising results

were compromised by signal weaknesses in both the design and the execution of his trials, while modern researchers generally agree that live vaccines of "wild" cultures are the most potent. In Spain, Ferrán is a medical hero. Elsewhere it is Haffkine who dominates histories of cholera vaccine; the rare accounts that mention Ferrán refer to his "injudicious" actions.

Another product of the laboratory was cholera's cure. Here the story was a sort of comedy: the end product of high science was common sense. Saline therapies are the keystone of the modern therapy for cholera and other severe diarrheas. Often rehydration is all that is necessary. In serious cases saline will be given intravenously, but oral rehydration is normally enough. It has seemed ironic that so devastating a disease as cholera can be cured by simple means that lay persons may easily learn to administer. It has also seemed puzzling that it should have taken a century and a half to discover these simple truths. Once oral rehydration therapy had been recognized, there was some interest in rereading the history of cholera therapy to find that it had been there all along. As I noted in Chapter 1, it had been; though among much else.

One job of historians of science is to explain why what seems obvious was not. For rehydration, that is hard. Most cholera— though importantly, not all—was plainly a process of massive fluid loss. Surely that fluid came from somewhere inside a hitherto healthy body; seemingly recovery would require its replacement. Loss of fluid clearly affected blood. Cholera blood was black and thick. It also differed in composition and was deficient in some of the "saline" constituents of normal blood. Surely no advanced degree was needed to appreciate these relations.

Indeed, all this was plain, at least to some of the observers of the Moscow epidemics in 1830–1. Injection of saline solutions was famously proposed in 1832 by William O'Shaughnessy and tried by the young Edinburgh practitioner Thomas Latta. It was seen by most to have failed, but was repeatedly tried, and repeatedly failed. Only around 1910 did it begin to become commonplace in India, through the work of the Anglo-Indian pathologist (not, importantly, a clinician) Leonard Rogers. Rogers's approach was initially a laboratory one. It was based on a theorized body quantitatively translated into physical parameters of blood. It cut cholera mortality to a third of what it had been, yet would be recognized as based on an erroneous theory. In the 1960s, new practices based in new theories would cut cholera mortality by two orders of magnitude or more.

But why did it take so long even to get to Rogers? A few factors—theoretical, practical, empirical—may help suspend some disbelief, if not all. Theory first. Older theories of cholera had often represented fluid loss as desirable or incidental. As noted earlier, the old *cholera morbus* was a humoral disease. Cholera was the body's expulsion of bile; the vomiting and diarrhea were not inherently pathological, but restorative. Cholera was a dangerous rite of passage requiring medical supervision, but the body was merely undergoing seasonal readjustment or responding to indigestible foods or other ill-defined influences. In non-humoral theories of cholera—those preoccupied with its spasms, or treating it as a kind of blood poisoning—fluid loss might be incidental. It would go away when the underlying causes were addressed.

Yet this is not explanation enough: that most cholera clinicians did see fluid loss as secondary to some other malign process need not disguise its dangerousness. Most cholera therapies were geared to addressing several problems simultaneously; it is not clear why rehydration should not have been among them more often.

There were practical problems. There are two main ways to rehydrate: orally and hypodermically, whether into a vein or simply through skin. Always, vomiting was the fatal flaw in oral rehydration. (Modern clinical discussions often downplay vomiting, representing it as an occasional early symptom whose role in cholera is not well understood. Clinicians are urged to keep giving liquids and fall back on intravenous administration if need be.)

Sticking people with needles, on the other hand, was not a common part of medical practice until the end of the nineteenth century. Needles were tools of experimental physiologists, and associated with the dubious heritage of transfusion.

And, finally, there was a long record of failure. Attempts at injecting fluid (usually subcutaneous) often produced remarkable but temporary improvement. Reminiscences, like this from Nelson, are Frankensteinesque:

> The moribund state of this strong man before the injection and his sudden apparent recovery gave to many of the bystanders the idea of a ghostly resurrection of a corpse; some of them left the room in terror. In me it excited the sentiment of a total refutation of the doctrines of physiology—a dead man brought back to life, as it were, by merely filling the vessels with a fluid not natural to the body. The heat was once more set agoing, and a feeble pulse could be felt at the wrist; the mind once more restored—some thought. Can a recently dead man be restored to life…[27]

Yet patients soon relapsed; mortality rates (based on small numbers and often severe cases) were sometimes worse than the pathetic rates for less dramatic therapies. Rogers calculated an 84 percent mortality rate for the Edinburgh trials of Latta and Mackintosh in 1832. As Michael Durey points out, the rejection of saline injection exhibits the proper operation of scientific

method: "it was the same rigorous demand for empirical confirmation of theory which led to the demise of *both* potentially
useful *and* potentially dangerous therapies."[28]

Marked improvements and obviousness were reason enough
to keep trying. But, beyond the incidental problems that arose
from lack of sterility and other problems of injection, the grand
problem was that there was no adequate guide for determining
how much to inject, and of what. That inadequacy is only apparent retrospectively. For, at each stage, it finally seemed clear that
enough was known about cholera, fluids, and blood to make
the program work. To us, the efforts seem appallingly trial-and-
error. Roughly there were two approaches, one focusing more
on composition, the delivery of missing substances, the other
on concentration, matters of the physical chemistry of flow
across membranes. Both mattered; only in the 1950s would they
be adequately joined.

Rogers provides a good axis both for what precedes and for
what follows. If, for many impecunious British doctors, the
Indian Medical Service (IMS) was a path to lucrative private
practice, for Rogers it was an opening to a career in laboratory
medicine. The facilities in Kolkata were adequate; there was a
teaching (and research) hospital, abject patients, and an abun-
dance of poorly understood tropical diseases. His cholera work
was but one of many projects. Rogers began studying cholera in
1902. His first concern was systematic study of the changes in
the choleraic blood. He was looking at specific gravity and at the
only recently quantified parameter of blood pressure, but also
at the concentration of solid contents—red and white corpus-
cles. Rogers suspected that earlier rehydration experimenters
had not given enough fluid. Knowing precisely how much each
individual had lost would be the key to better therapy. Use of

this precision rehydration approach brought a slight improvement of mortality rates. By 1907, Rogers was thinking more in terms of concentrations. Higher concentrations of salts in the blood might aid in fluid retention; perhaps what mattered was less the right amount of diluting fluid than ebb and flow across membranes. He began trying as much as twice the previous dose of sodium chloride in a hypertonic saline solution (most earlier versions had been modestly hypotonic). This produced a rapid drop in mortality, to under a third.

Rogers felt he had solved the main problem of cholera therapy. In the next decade he addressed two of the proximate causes of cholera deaths: fever and uremia. Attributing fever to the continued toxic effects of the vibrio, he added potassium permanganate, which would kill the bugs, to the rehydrant solution. The uremia, he learned from others' researches, was tied to acidification of the blood and could be combated by adding sodium bicarbonate to the saline solutions. By around 1920 cholera mortality at the teaching hospital had dropped to about 20 percent and Rogers had moved on to other challenges.

Rogers represented his achievement as the difference that the systematic approach of the pathologist could make in clinical practice—which, he hints, had been but the repetition of traditional remedies by a succession of *Indian* house officers. And yet, as a pathologist, Rogers was largely self-taught. To any properly pedigreed German researcher he would have seemed a Kolkatan Ferrán. His experimental work was trivial, and his knowledge of the field slight, even appalling. What Rogers enjoyed, much more than Ferrán, was freedom to fail. Both exploited the rising reputation of laboratory medicine that the profound achievements of German and French laboratories were underwriting, while following their own independent paths. Both found freedom to act in conditions of desperation and of minimal medical oversight, though Ferrán, clinician first and researcher second, living in a constitutional democracy, was subject to much more scrutiny than the researcher Rogers, who had the advantage of being a colonizer studying the colonized.

When, in the 1950s, teams of American cholera researchers arrived in Dhaka and Kolkata, it was in a neocolonial context, the cold-war courting of south Asian affections. They found Rogers's rule of hypertonic saline still being followed. Yet the careful quantification and supplementary use of permanganate and bicarbonate had not been kept up. Cholera mortality had climbed back to 30 percent.

But their critique was not only of complacency in clinical management; Rogers too, they concluded, had been insufficiently critical toward his own findings. He had been wrong about the need for hypertonic solutions. Too much and too concentrated fluid could lead to pulmonary edema, another common cause of cholera mortality. More generally, preoccupied with saline *concentrations*, Rogers had failed to give sufficient attention to composition, in particular to potassium loss. A better way to chart the changes cholera produced in the body was to analyze the stool, not the blood. They developed a new strategy of rehydration: injection of isotonic saline, replacement of potassium, and continued monitoring of blood pH. This quickly brought mortality down to 5 percent, and eventually to under 1 percent.

None of these factors was wholly novel. Others had supplemented sodium chloride with potassium chloride, appreciated the problem of acid blood and used sodium bicarbonate against it, or seen the need for an ongoing saline drip and for the administration of large quantities commensurate with fluid loss. Greater familiarity with the full literature on clinical use of saline solutions might have led Rogers to fuller appreciation of some of these issues; yet equally they might have persuaded him that the full range of saline therapies had been tried and had failed.

It is indeed the case that, in the many rehydration experiments over the course of the nineteenth century, the obvious formulae will have been tried on one occasion or another. Primarily what changed was not the discovery of new constituents of blood or new ways to measure them, or recognition of the physiological states of edema or acidosis. Instead, what changed was confidence in laboratory medicine: a growing view that the relevant variables were finite in number and could be recognized and controlled, and ultimately that cholera was a lawful physical system. That confidence, if not fully founded, is evident in Rogers and even more so in the interdisciplinary teams of medical scientists sent by the American government to Asia in the 1950s.

Whether that confidence was shared by cholera victims had not mattered. It is hard to avoid a sense that lives in India were cheap. In such places, it had been and would be possible to do large-scale experiments on populations that were both exposed and tractable. Such trials would have been problematic in Europe or America (ironically, where informed confidence in scientific medicine was presumably higher). There was little accountability in these colonial clinical settings. But freedom to fail was also freedom to succeed. Even Rogers, one might argue, had not given himself enough freedom to fail. He had accepted as a relative success what his successors would see as unnecessary failure.

Confident that they could restore the body's equilibrium with intravenous solutions, the American experts were much

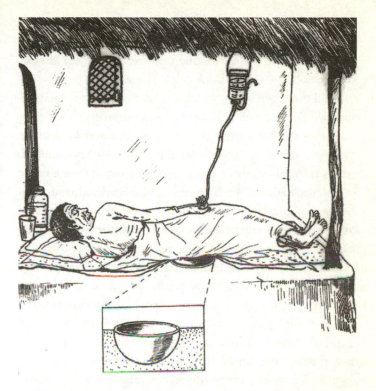

15. This drawing from the 1970s reflects the combination of high tech medicine in low tech settings; here the combined use of IV rehydration in a hut, with a hole underneath the bowels to collect involuntary rice-water discharges. Cots with such holes would become a standard means of maintaining cleanliness of bedding in cholera treatment. (*Burrows and Barua, Cholera, 1974*)

less confident that the same salts could be introduced orally. Beyond the practical problem of vomiting was a physiological one: most of the restorative ions would cross from the gut into the body, but the crucial sodium would not—unless, noticed Howard Phillips, it was accompanied by glucose.

Yet even after the glucose breakthrough in the late 1950s, and even in cases where vomiting was manageable, there remained great unease with oral rehydration. To some it seemed impossible that saline could be drunk quickly enough. The perspective reflected how far-reaching had been the triumph of laboratory medicine. The recovery of health required conceiving the human being as controlled system. To trust the mouth, and the absorption by the unruly gut over the needle seemed unduly chancy, a willing relinquishment of power and precision. It took a crisis even to demonstrate the feasibility of oral rehydration: during the 1971 war that led to formation of Bangladesh, there was too little intravenous saline; but the requisite salts for oral intake could be made up quickly in large quantities. And they worked.

These were key stages on what may be called the de-medicalization of cholera therapy. By the 1990s, it would be noted that the pure and relatively costly glucose was not essential; other sugars and easily digested carbohydrates—rice, for example—conveyed sodium too. Intense thirst is a frequent theme in nineteenth-century cholera accounts; clinicians anguish about whether any drink can be safely given. That thirst would now be trusted; oral rehydrants were to be available *ad libitum*. Unneeded salts would simply pass through. Family members need not be kept from the bedside; they were the ideal persons to provide the drink or mild foods.

Cholera anatomized

Outside India, chiefly in Europe, post-Koch cholera science had turned to the laboratory and the animal model. Initially the domain of bacteriology, cholera science would migrate as bacteriology evolved into immunology, immunology into biochemistry, then into molecular genetics. Ultimately some would escape, returning to the field as a branch of ecology. For most of the period, epidemiology would be marginalized, serving simply as a way to test bacteriological hypotheses. With the fading of Pettenkoferianism, the long heritage of geographic studies would be forgotten, only to be rediscovered in the first decade of the twenty-first century.

In the early years of the twentieth century the quantity of cholera research remained prodigious. But it slowly fell—especially in parts of the world that saw themselves as unthreatened by cholera. By the mid 1950s the community of American cholera researchers could meet in a hotel room, note Van Henyigen and Seal. The seventh pandemic, beginning in 1961, together with greater funding and newly exploitable techniques, brought a new wave of research. The best gauge of changing issues and approaches are the occasional cholera compendia. The greatest was Pollitzer's. He could compile because cholera seemed largely a matter of the past. Yet the seventh pandemic and revolutions in cholera therapeutics and toxicology in the 1950s and 1960s would quickly make vast sections of the great work obsolete. Subsequent compendia would be edited compilations of chapters by specialist authors. The first, by Dhiman Barua and William Burrows, would come out in 1974. The return of cholera to the Americas in the early 1990s and its becoming endemic in sub-Saharan Africa led to another round of compendia. But the years since have seen enormous shifts in the content and agenda of cholera science. Renewed interest in what *Vibrio cholerae* is up to at all those times when it is not infesting humans arose with growing recognition that a changing climate would surely shift the character and distribution of infectious diseases.

Around 1900, at the beginning of this scientific age of cholera, the key focus of research was the distinctiveness of the comma bacillus. Because the bacillus was defined as the cause of cholera, that research would also, incidentally, address the question that Koch had largely ducked: how it killed. Edward Klein was one of many to raise the problem of the specificity of Koch's microbe. Comma-shaped microbes were common, he insisted. Some were harmful. Koch's claim that he had seen them *only* in association with cholera cases suggested to Klein a distressing unfamiliarity with the microscopic world. At issue was the applicability of the species concept. Klein and many English colleagues were intrigued—even besotted—by the doctrine of pleomorphism: in classifying bacteria one did not trust shape; it might be an artifact of environment. There might be only a few basic types with highly variable appearance.

Koch agreed that, in classifying bacteria, it was not possible to rely on shape alone. But he did trust behavior in culture. Each species would respond in a unique way to a combination of growth media and physical conditions—thus the comma bacillus liquefied gelatine in a different pattern from other similarly shaped organisms. Growing cultures in a range of media would allow one to create a unique profile for each species, which would in turn serve to define that species as the entity that exhibited that composite of cultural characteristics. Yet one might also hope to hit on a simple diagnostic test. From the 1880s into the 1930s there was interest in a so-called "cholera red" reaction: sulfuric acid, added to a cholera culture, produced a reddish tinge. Later it would be in the Voges–Proskauer reaction, in which a combination of α-naphthol, potassium hydroxide, and creatine are added to a culture in a glucose broth, which turns pinkish in the presence of *Vibrio cholerae* (but also some other species).

But the most powerful means of distinguishing bacteria were not artificial media, but animal immune systems. By the mid 1890s, a new science of serology had emerged, the achievement largely of Richard Pfeiffer, a student of Koch's. When blood serum from an animal that had been injected or exposed to a particular microbe was added to a culture of that microbe, the cells would agglutinate. Pfeiffer was recognizing antigenic specificity. Antigen molecules trigger the host's production of antibodies, immune system agents that will then target any microbes containing the antigen. During the 1930s, the O antigen, a portion of lipopolysaccharide in the cell membrane of *Vibrio cholerae*, would become the most important.

But the O antigen turned out to be not one, but many. Among the varieties included within it was a microbe found at the Suez quarantine station at El Tor in 1905. The disease it produced was milder, yet, being hardier than Koch's variety, the El Tor microbe seemed likely to be important in spreading a cholera-like disease. Was that disease cholera? To those who equated "cholera" with the disease caused by Koch's microbe, it could not be. "Paracholera" might be a better term, clinically justifiable because the disease was milder. The El Tor microbe had the ability to lyse blood cells, which Koch's microbe did not; that seemed important. Yet, serologically, the El Tor variant would be included not only within the species *Vibrio cholerae*, but also within the O1 serogroup, where it coexisted with the so-called classical O1, Koch's microbe. It would ultimately be recognized as *Vibrio cholerae* O1, biotype eltor, cause of a real cholera.

Research to track down all the varieties of *Vibrio cholerae* occupied the better part of a century. Figures for how many serogroups (types of O antigen) of *Vibrio cholerae* there are vary from 139 to "around 200." By the late 1930s serogroups had been supplemented by classification in terms of one of three pre-sumably stable serotypes (or serovars), designated after their discoverers as Inaba, Ogawa, and Hirojima. Until 1993, only *Vibrio cholerae* O1 was seen to cause epidemic cholera. Others were diarrhea-producers, but these "non-O1" *Vibrio cholerae* were rarely cultured for and were generally dismissed as "environmental" variants. In that year a second epidemic-producing serotype, O139, would be found responsible for outbreaks in Bengal.

Yet, in the long term, serological distinctions proved unsat-isfactory as the master set of taxonomic criteria. There were many problems. Most importantly, the possession of common antigens did not imply common everything else: there was both great variability within antigenic categories and simi-larity across them. Arriving in the 1980s, the powerful tools of molecular genetics would bring new ways to classify. One would speak of ribovars, based on characteristic stretches of DNA. These new analytical abilities would underwrite a new regime of molecular epidemiology. Having multiple genetic markers made it much clearer how a particular strain of cholera had spread. Yet they did not bring unanimity on the broader question of how to understand differences among the many varieties of *Vibrio cholerae*. Different analytic procedures gave different breakdowns. The fallback was simply to work out empirical clusters of characteristics that a particular strain exhibited, and to give up trying to explain the possession of such characteristics in ulterior terms.

There had been hope that greater taxonomic precision would clarify what was so deadly about *Vibrio cholerae* O1. To under-stand the differences among types of *Vibrio cholerae* in terms of antigens reflected how far the vibrio had come to be defined

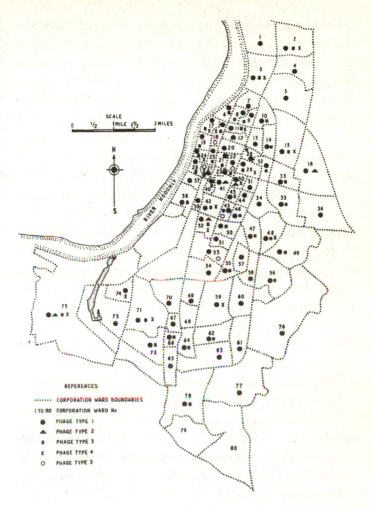

16. The multiplicity of new techniques for distinguish strains of *Vibrio cholerae* has allowed the development of molecular epidemiology, which makes possible much more precise tracking of the movement of epidemics – here in Kolkota. The technique here is a relatively early version, based on differential susceptibility to various phages. (*Burrows and Barua, Cholera, 1974*)

in terms of its effects on humans. Biologically, such molecules had no inherent importance to the organisms thatpossessed them; they were simply flags that others species happened to recognize.

Not only were pathological microbes being seen as essentially pathological; what was biologically distinct about them was being expected to mirror what was pathologically distinct. Classification based on antigens was compelling because it seemed possible that comprehending the antigenic profile of the single deadly variant of the cholera vibrio would shed light on *how* it did its deadly work. How convenient it would be if the antigens that called forth immune response were the same as, or intimately related to, whatever it was that harmed the host.

That seductive assumption was little challenged for the first half of the twentieth century. Surely higher organisms could be trusted to have evolved to finger precisely the elements of invading microbes that made them sick. It turned out to be a gratuitous assumption: that one part of a pathogenic microbe happened to alert a host's immune system had nothing necessarily to do with the havoc being wreaked by another part.

In the case of cholera, this gratuitous assumption was to hold sway into the 1960s. It was part of a broader misunderstanding about what cholera did to the human body. Though its agent entered by mouth and multiplied in the gut, Koch, like most of his colleagues, had assumed that cholera was a systemic disease. After all, its manifestations were throughout the body: in spasms, in fever, in effects on heart and kidney function. It was easy to imagine that the microbe irritated the lining of the gut, which both let the body's fluids flow out and let the microbe and its poisonous products in to spread throughout the system.

The assumption could be tested. Inject cholera bacteria or cell-free filtrates of it into a vein, muscle, or the abdominal cavity and there will probably be some kind of pathological response. The experimental animal may die. The assumption was that it was dying in the same way it would have done had the cholera poison reached it naturally, spreading out over the body from the small intestine. Koch and his successors were assuming that cholera's toxic effect was due to an endotoxin, a substance within a microbe that was released or activated as that microbe succumbed to the body's defenses. *Vibrio cholerae*, like many other microbes, has endotoxins. They do sometimes kill. They trigger the immune response to the vibrio; they were the basis of Ferrán's and Haffkine's vaccines, but they do *not* produce clinical cholera. Van Henyigen and Seal sum up the decades of misdirection in no uncertain terms: "The wrong material was administered by the wrong route by the wrong people, and practically every experiment was worthless as far as cholera was concerned."[29] Too many had made the gratuitous assumption.

The toxin that did produce those effects began to be recognized and isolated only at the end of the 1950s in separate ways in two Indian laboratories. Best known is the rabbit ileal loop experiment of S. N. De of Kolkata. It was a simple experiment, an adaptation of a line of exploration that had been taken up and dropped a half century earlier. The ileum—a section of small intestine—was closed off at each end. A cell-free filtrate of *Vibrio cholerae* was injected. The section was soon swollen with fluid. Plainly this chemical substance was pulling water across the ileal wall, producing what would have been, had the ileum not been closed off, the rice-water diarrhea of cholera. So strongly held was belief in cholera as a systemic endotoxic

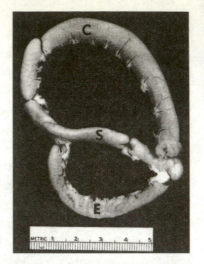

17 De's discovery of the cholera toxin relied on the swelling of a length of rabbit small intestine, ligatured at both ends, when injected with a cell-free cholera extract. Here section C shows the swelling due to cholera. (*Burrows and Barua, Cholera, 1974*)

disease, that the implication—that one was looking here at the main toxic process of cholera—was initially unclear.

During the 1960s the composition and structure of this cholera toxin (Ctx) would be worked out; so too in later decades would be the mechanism of its operation. It was, in the first place, an exotoxin, emitted by the microbe in certain circumstances. It did not act by destroying any part of the intestinal wall. The long history of observations of intestinal inflammation, the occasional finding of *Vibrio cholerae* in various bodily cavities, were ultimately reinterpreted as post-mortem artifacts. As Klein had warned, however tempting it might be to read lesions found upon autopsy as consequences of pathological processes in the living body, it was unwarranted: even if they were unique to cholera, they might be due simply to post-mortem decomposition. The discovery made sense of all manner of anomalies in earlier experiments: it explained, for example, why the symptoms from the injection of cholera cultures often bore little resemblance to clinical cholera.

The new cholera toxin would be shown to have two quite different components. Component "A" did the actual damage. It interacted with cells that lined the intestine to alter the operation of one of the body's principal energy release processes, that of cyclic AMP. cAMP moved chlorine ions across the membrane, through the mucus layer and out into the intestinal channel; sodium, potassium, and water went with them. But in the presence of the cholera toxin, a process that was ordinarily regulated by a complicated feedback became nonstop. Surrounding that "A" component were five "B" units, binding the toxin to the intestinal lining. That compound toxin would turn out not to be unique to cholera. As a common enterotoxin, it, or its analogues, would be found in some strains of *Escherichia coli*, most common of the coliform bacteria, and a microbe long considered innocuous. And, while it was known for its work in the gut, it could carry out its actions on any sort of cell.

It was possession of this toxin that would distinguish O1 from non-O1 *Vibrio cholerae*. Or so it seemed at first. Beginning in the 1980s, it became ever easier to scan for certain genes. There were surprises. Non-O1 *Vibrio cholerae* sometimes had the toxin; O1 sometimes did not. It became possible to determine what those genes did by introducing strains from which they had been removed. It was found that the mere possession of the genes for the toxin was not enough; something had to cause their expression, and also that O1 still caused diarrhea *after* removal of the toxin.

Resolving these anomalies revealed an ever more complicated cholera process, involving supplemental toxins and complementary toxin-activating elements. The mechanisms of colonization of the gut and of the mooring of the toxin at the edge of the intestinal epithelium became clearer. The vibrio propelled itself with its flagellum, steering by chemical signals. On approaching the jagged coastline of the intestinal wall, it released proteolytic enzymes to ease passage through the mucosal swamps. It then released chemicals to prepare for infection. Some of these agglutinated the blood cells, others prepared the gangliosides in epithelial cells to dock with the toxin's B subunit, still others were the accessory toxins, ZOT ("zonal occlusion toxin") and ACE ("accessory cholera enterotoxin").[30] Still other substances would allow operation in an environment of limited iron. By the early 1990s a new and hitherto under-recognized component of this process was being recognized: the eruption from *Vibrio cholerae* of pili, of which it carried three types. These thin strands of protein converged into a stalk-like appendage that was crucial in that anchoring. One is tempted to imagine the alien toxin commandos leaving the vibrio mothership and crawling down the pilus to undertake their dirty deeds on a shore that has already been softened up and prepared by sappers and miners. (In fact, it is not clear that the pilus functions in quite that way.) Yet to call all this, as some have done, cholera's "infection strategy" certainly seems apt.[31]

The sequencing of an El Tor genome, completed in 2000, opened the door to exploration of *Vibrio cholerae*'s two chromosomes. The larger and more stable has been dubbed the "core" or the "ancestral chromosome."[32] The smaller was the site of greater variability. One of the gene clusters found there—or gene islands, chips, packages, cassettes (the metaphors came, like many in genetics, from computer science as well as from geography)—was known as "vibrio pathogenicity island" (VPI). Various strains of cholera contained one, two, or three copies of this cluster: El Tor had one, classical two, and O139, the new strain of the 1990s, three. But sometimes it was absent.

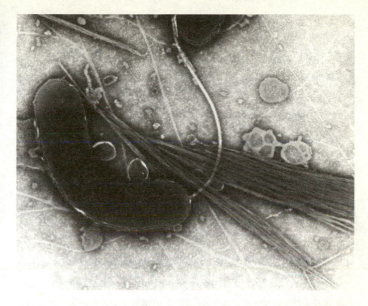

18. The 'comma' bacillus with long flagellum and pili. (*Louisa Howard, Dartmouth College*)

By the 1990s it was becoming clear that *one* reason it was so hard to classify *Vibrio cholerae* was that it was not a stable entity. Its identity varied with environment. There were claims that agglutination specificity, so central in identifying varieties of *Vibrio cholerae*, was not fixed. Nor was hemolysis a fixed characteristic for distinguishing "classical" from "eltor" (the former could gain it; the latter could lose it). Inaba could change to Ogawa. Much of this had been reported much earlier. The reports had been disregarded, or grudgingly accepted, but not allowed to threaten orthodoxy. Limited variability might be accommodated within a framework dominated by the concept of species and the expectation of stability.

Yet from early on in the bacteriological age it had been clear that microbes not only transformed their media but were also significantly transformed by them. Pasteur had relied on such transformations to attenuate virulence, and thus develop vaccines. Failure to replicate some experimental result had often been attributed to a culture being "old," even though it had continually been replanted in fresh media (the equivalent, presumably, of having its cage cleaned). In some cases it seemed important that a culture periodically be taken from glassware to pass through an animal, as a sort of revivifying holiday. Often it would be claimed that *in vitro* was no adequate indication of *in vivo*, though this rarely stopped reliance on *in vitro* techniques, which were so much easier. *V. cholerae* 569 B was the best toxin producer, but only *in vitro*. Toxin production *in vitro* was affected by shaking a culture—how was that to translate to living bodies? It is only in retrospect that we can see the cup as half-empty rather than half-full: the evidence of variability seems overwhelming, and much greater than that for stability.

The variability would turn out to be far more radical than Klein and the English pleomorphists had ever imagined. It would have horrified Koch. In 1996 Matthew Waldor and John Melankanos reported that Ctx was in no sense inherent to *Vibrio cholerae*.[33] It came from a virus, a filamentous phage designated CTX-Φ, through a horizontal gene transfer process. The process was not an unusual one in the microbial world; decades earlier it had become clear that microbe species were sharing genes for antibiotic resistance. Yet the detailing of cholera's genome had diverted attention from the question of where bits of its genetic material might be coming from. Soon it would be found that other bits were coming from outside too. Far from being the distinct and stable species Koch had imagined, microbes were polymorphous perverts, hooking up—sometimes by their pili—with other microbes, opening themselves to viruses.

How could this postmodern *Vibrio cholerae*, lacking any clear identity, really be responsible for the disease cholera, if it was not responsible for itself, but was rather the site of accidental transformations, as "packages" of DNA moved readily from strain to strain and species to species? Even its pathogenicity, its most important quality from a human vantage point, was one of these accidents. Some *Vibrio cholerae* were inadvertent carriers of dangerous genes, just like the naive air passenger, duped into carrying some terrorist's deadly tools. A few of these then chanced to end up in the bowels of undernourished Bangladeshi children with insufficiently acid stomachs, where some incidental combination of factors ignited those bombs. Not only could *Vibrio cholerae* not be blamed, except for naivety or excess promiscuity; neither could CTX-Φ: the toxin gene cluster had no essential use for it either.

Yet what Waldor and Melakanos found did not quite fit this scenario either. Competing with the image of the postmodern microbe was that of shrewd and adaptive enemy. For the transfer of the toxin package from CTX-Φ to *Vibrio cholerae* did not occur randomly. It took place only where *Vibrio cholerae* already possessed another gene essential to the pathological process, TcpA, the toxin coregulating pilus gene, which launched the stalk-like pilus. Moreover, that transfer was likelier to occur in a site of potential pathogenic activity, like the bowel of a mouse, than in a laboratory setting. "The phage appears to be 'choosing' a bacterium that is able to express Ct," wrote two reviewers.[34]

Far from randomness and innocence, here were resonances of malignity. The production of toxicity, it turned out, required a cascade of events, with one set of genes, under particular environmental conditions, turning on another set, and then another, and so forth. The VPI alone could not make the microbe toxic. Genes from the "ancestral" chromosome were deeply implicated. Microscopists had often been fascinated by the grace of mitosis or meiosis; here was a courtly dance between the dowager ancestral chromosome and the more recent and variable partner: teenage genetic riff-raff in for the weekend. AphA and AphB, genes on the ancestral chromosome, activated TcpP on the VPI on the smaller chromosome. Then TcpP and ToxR (ancestral) together activated ToxT on the island, ToxT activated Acf, and the Ctx on the CTX-Φ.

Who was responsible for all this? Whose agenda was being consummated in what two researchers described as a "series of horizontal gene transfers that allowed a benign marine bacterium to rapidly evolve into a dangerous human pathogen"? Was TcpA on the look out for rogue toxins to complete its insidious design; or, alternatively, did the toxin, to consummate its own purposes, seek out maidenly TcpA to seduce? Or, worse, was the attraction mutual, a true conspiracy? Moreover, one could not assume that these relationships were stable: "V. Cholerae continues to evolve as a human pathogen."[35]

The complicated expression of the genes of toxicity, including the Eisenhoweresque landing on the beaches of the small bowel, may easily be seen as "tactical" achievements, but were they truly strategic as well? Here, too, the representation of genetic processes and of microbes as somehow the dumb agents of nature not nurture had changed. The old "central dogma" of biology of the 1960s and 1970s—DNA makes RNA makes proteins—had broken down utterly. Genomes did not blindly and stupidly manufacture identical proteins to carry out the same operations. In 1990s lingo, pathological agents like *Vibrio cholerae* were smart weapons or shrewd entrepreneurs; they sensed changes in the environment, and retooled.

One might well worry that toxic action in the human gut was indeed somehow part of the cholera business plan, yet, at the same time, most *Vibrio cholerae*, those little-studied 198 other biotypes, did not usually have the toxin gene, or, if they did, did not (or could not?) use it. Yet the fact that expression of toxicity was greatest at 30 degrees celsius, somewhat cooler than the human small bowel, seemed significant: perhaps even they were only accidental offenders.

Cholera's vivisectors had given it their best shot. They had plucked out genes and molecules with their wee tweezers and put them in their little jars, only to have their subject pop up, smile, and, with a friendly "F*** You," go on about their business.

As noted in Chapter 2, for many people during the nineteenth century, the great question about cholera was not how but why? Plainly it was our enemy, but what were its goals? Was it out to kill us all, perhaps as God's retributive agent, or to prod or test us, as God's redemptive motor, as Kingsley and Acland believed, or did it just have its own amoral Darwinian ends? Kochian microbiology had buried such questions: the pathogenicity of some microbes for some species was one of those things that just happened to be the case—primarily, one hoped to show which species did it, and how they might be stopped. How pathogenicity worked was a barely recognized question; why it should exist was hopelessly metaphysical. The practical approach accomplished a great deal: cholera was exiled from the developed world; elsewhere it represented the willful failure to develop or be developed.

I have turned off the analogy-creating censors in the last few pages to make a point. All this is, arguably, uncharacteristic of modern science; it is not merely speculation, but something worse, use of language that dispenses with caution and precision in pursuit of meaning-making. Yet it is also the addressing of questions that many people continue to ask about infectious and other diseases. Auguste Comte put the stage of meaning-making before the stage of positive knowledge. Facts are to drive out meanings. They do not. Cholera is as meaning packed now as ever it was.

VI

⧪

CHOLERA'S LAST LAUGH

I n 1991 cholera popped up in the western hemisphere for the first time in more than a century. Beginning in coastal Peru, it overspread most of the continent, and moved northward into Mexico. A handful of food-borne or travellers' cases occurred in the USA. In most places the response was rapid and effective. And yet the familiar pattern of spread was proof that scientific sophistication and extraordinary technical power were ill-matched where the problems were poverty or even racism. Cholera can now be cured and prevented. One may ask why it is not always prevented and why rates of cure are uneven. Such questions take us back to earlier eras; they are central themes of cholera's history.

Histories of cholera exist in reciprocal relation with science. Cholera scientists and practitioners invoke conceptions of cholera's past; historians make contemporary knowledge of cholera the fulcrum of their explanations of its past. But there may be lag times, when one enterprise is out of phase with the other. Knowledge of cholera is changing quickly; new findings invite a new history, which will feed back on how we think about cholera in the present.

These changes prompt the old saw about "the more things change..." In many ways what cholera is now is what it was in 1830: a severe diarrhea, one of many; a concomitant of poverty. But the way back to simplicity has come through complexity. Cholera, so painstakingly pinned down by Koch, is again inchoate. It is even defined differently in different contexts. Questions that had animated nineteenth-century researchers—for example, of the geography and periodicity of outbreaks—are again central.

In particular, cholera

- may not be (or may not always have been) a south Asian export;
- is caused by a group of genetically unstable organisms, whose main ecological niche is warm seas not the human intestine;
- is, as a clinical matter, indistinct from other severe diarrheas (including the old *cholera nostras*) and is often defined in clinical rather than bacteriological terms;
- is subject to seasonal and environmental factors, not merely to the presence of infected persons;
- is not exclusively, or often even predominantly, water-borne, and may not always be a fecal–oral disease;
- is as much a political problem as ever.

In most respects, "cholera" is fuzzier than it was in the confident 1950s when Pollitzer wrote. Certainly much more is known about it. Only rarely does the new knowledge drive out the older; it does show it as oversimplified. And there is less certainty.

What is cholera really?

Reinterpretation of cholera's history has implications for modern treatment, diagnosis, and prevention. Recognition of a distinct Asiatic cholera in the 1830s required that the disease that broke out in India around 1817 be fundamentally different from a disease long known in Europe. A view would develop that cholera had always been in south Asia, periodically culling the population, and that it had, possibly, increased in frequency or virulence in the late eighteenth century. A corollary was that the "cholera" of pre-nineteenth-century Europe was something else, and probably no single disease. Occasional dissent had been founded in skepticism. Clinically, sometimes even epidemiologically, what had been called cholera in Europe was indistinguishable from Asian cholera. The view of the comma bacillus as indigenous to India might have been true for the twentieth century, but we could not be sure about earlier times. Repeated in text after text, the view of cholera as uniquely and eternally "Asiatic" gelled into fact.

Yet, already in 1925, the eminent Anglo-Indian cholera epidemiologist A. J. R. Russell had worried about "the custom blindly to transfer a statement made by one author into succeeding volumes or papers on the same subject ... [when] careful scrutiny frequently reveals the original opinion to have been based on very doubtful evidence."[1] But Russell could not stop it. Pollitzer drew on Macnamara via Hirsch; most later writers drew on Pollitzer. Along the way, the cardinal rule of cholera epidemiology became "Cherchez l'Indien." In that received view, we could not have cholera without somebody being responsible for it; the search for cholera index cases became disturbingly resonant to witch-hunts.

That older view is not necessarily wrong. It can be supplemented with new knowledge. But it is possible and has become increasingly plausible to read these facts differently, and to see better how the older view might have seemed especially plausible in a colonial era. Where Howard-Jones was adamant, modern authorities either are more cautious, or draw the opposite conclusion. Descriptions of seventeenth- and eighteenth-century European cholera "indicate that *cholera morbus* was no different from true cholera, having the same potential to cause epidemics," one modern authority writes.[2]

That perspective represents a shift in the burden of proof that comes with a different contextual landscape. One may argue that the ability to cure cholera lessens the importance of constraining it to a single site of origin and pronouncing definitively on its means of transfer. That ability, and greater appreciation of the many factors determining cholera's incidence, can make us comfortable with less certainty. Inability to reduce an outbreak to a single route of transmission need not paralyze our ability to respond effectively.[3]

In this new knowledge-rich domain what were once anomalies reappear as interesting research questions. Could it be that some cholera outbreaks were and are truly local? Historically, the charting of cholera's pandemics had been central to the conviction of its transmissibility, and tied to its Indian origin (all but the seventh, which came from Sulawesi, started when cholera left India). Pandemic mongering is essentially an empirical operation: date the outbreak of cholera in particular places and draw arrows from earlier to later using rules of proximity or of known routes of contact. The chief induction from such exercises, that cholera always came from somewhere, was usually an assumption. It was asserted also that cholera never traveled faster than humans, and always broke out in the nearer place before the further. Usually one could make such patterns. Given a long enough span, the likelihood was high that a place where cholera broke out had been in contact with a place where it had previously been. But what was the permissible lag time between supposed transmission and evident outbreak? And what of places, like Bengal, where cholera flared up everywhere all at once?

More or less grudgingly, Pollitzer, and before him Hirsch, had acknowledged the phenomenon of "recrudescence." Cholera's agent or essence had somehow stayed in a region from an earlier pandemic, either in the environment or persisting as sporadic or asymptomatic cases within a large host population. Then, for some reason, it was reactivated as part of a subsequent pandemic. Disagreements about which outbreaks were importations and which were recrudescences account for much of the disagreement about how to count cholera pandemics. Yet getting the number right had not affected the overarching generalization that sooner or later all cholera had come from India. And, always, recrudescence was a conclusion of exhaustion, a possibility to be entertained only after ruling out all plausible routes of transmission.

But might the exception be the rule; the noise, the signal? In the 1990s some cholera experts were beginning to wonder if perhaps cholera had been in place all along. Perhaps the concept of recrudescence, based on the presumption of earlier importation, was misconceived. This new possibility reflected converging ecological studies, which revealed that *Vibrio cholerae* was widely distributed in nature.

That new picture of the natural history of cholera had begun to emerge in the 1970s. It reflected the convergence of several research paths. On one hand was a long-standing frustration that *Vibrio cholerae*'s behavior in culture seemed so often not to match its behavior in nature. On the other was a growing record of its detection in oceans, estuaries, and rivers, and deepening concern with so-called environmental, non O1, *Vibrio cholerae varieties.* Distributed throughout the world, they were much more common than the pathogen O1. They were in seafood (oysters, crabs, prawns), but also in terrestrial animals, wild and domestic. They were sometimes evidently responsible for a seasonal (summer and fall) gastroenteritis. Sometimes the diarrhea they caused was severe, with 20–30 stools per day; it might appear as "a cholera-like disease with rice-water stools...clinically indistinguishable" from cholera, though usually it was less virulent and did not become epidemic. While there was no single mechanism of toxicity, a good many NCV and non-O1 cases (29 percent in one Bangladesh study) did possess the classical cholera toxin.[4]

As the powerful techniques of molecular epidemiology were brought to bear, it became clear that there were distinct regional varietals of *Vibrio cholerae* residing—who knew for how long—in various environmental niches, possessing pathological potential but rarely causing disease. A strain on the east coast of Australia was causing small outbreaks in the 1970s: these "may have existed in the Australian environment for eons," noted one epidemiologist. Another strain, an O1 classical Inaba, lived off the gulf coast of the United States. Using crabs as a vector, this caused two small outbreaks in Louisiana in 1978. These might have been the recrudescence of the cholera that had attacked New Orleans in 1832 or 1849, or it might have been there for millennia.[5] The new model *Vibrio cholerae* was an "abundant, naturally occurring component of freshwater, estuarine, and marine ecosystems worldwide."[6] By 2002 it was being appreciated that "Vibrios, including *V. cholerae,* can be found in virtually any coastal water body especially in the tropics and subtropics, when appropriate techniques are used."[7]

There was also accumulating evidence that *Vibrio cholerae* did possess a resting stage. When nutrients were scarce, it rolled itself into a ball and, effectively, turned itself off. In this state it could not be cultured, though it could be observed microscopically and distinguished biochemically. That cholera could hunker down for as long as need be could explain apparent recrudescence of an introduced microbe; it was also consistent with the occasional pathogenicity of a resident microbe.[8]

Or perhaps pathogenicity was an acquired state. Nontoxigenic vibrios were occasionally transforming into toxigenic *Vibrio cholerae* O1, especially in the neighborhood of human communities or even in the human gut. This would explain why it was much easier to find non-O1 vibrios in the environment. It had been customary from the 1930s onward to treat the Inaba and Ogawa serotypes as firm taxonomic categories. During the South American outbreak, the strain of infecting microbe changed from Inaba to Ogawa in seven months. The same phenomenon occurred in the bodies of individual cholera victims. A century earlier, English bacteriologists had made pleomorphism a mainstay of their attack on Koch. To him, it had represented anarchic and irresponsible skepticism, a crotchet whose indulgence undercut the very possibility of bacteriological knowledge. Here, raising its ugly head was a far deeper pleomorphism, change not merely of shape but of identity.

As gene-swapping became the rule not a rarity and toxigenic strains came to seem transitory phenomena, there was less reason to invoke Macnamara's dictum of eternal cholera, always epidemic in Bengal, even if the ancient eastern sages had forgotten to mention it. In six years, *Vibrio cholerae* O139, the new cholera of the 1990s, had produced six ribotypes and eleven toxin genotypes in India and Bangladesh.

The breaking-out of cholera on the west coast of South America in 1991, rather than in Brazil, where it might easily have been tied to importation from West Africa, came as a surprise. Some attributed it to the shrinking global village. They looked to shipping or to international air travel, just as those in the age of Koch had been ready to blame steam and Suez. Yet the simultaneous appearance in several Peruvian port cities, distant from one another, was hard to square with a model of communication. And both O1 and non-O1 *Vibrio cholerae* had been found offshore in Central and South America as early as 1978. Perhaps the singular strain that caused the South American outbreak had long been at home in the offshore waters; it might even, like Heyerdahl's Argonauts, have crossed the Pacific, and arisen as part of the 1991 El Niño.

The vibrios of the world's oceans were capable of arranging their own transport, because they traveled with zooplankton. Chemically bonded to the chitonous shells of copepods, they recycled minerals, scavenged nutrients from phytoplankton wastes. Though harmful to us, their toxin might serve other species: it might regulate sodium in the copepod gut. They changed form, depending on physical conditions and their own population density, shifting from a free-living stage to a protective biofilm. They were part of food chains; other bacterivores lived on them.

Cholera's ecology would shed light on its epidemicity—a subject long avoided by researchers owing to its association with reactionary Anglo-Indian localism. In Bangladesh, where annual outbreaks were being attributed to marine sources, their intensity was shown to correlate with plankton blooms, and hence to be tied to global climatic events such as ENSO, the El Niño southern oscillation. Armed with powerful tools for grinding data, modern researchers were recovering the Anglo-Indian agenda—of seeking laws for the timing and distribution of cholera, even while their presumably intricate mechanisms remained elusive. Some researchers returned to the great and despised works of Bryden and Bellew, the Indian records so laboriously collected during the nineteenth century.

Not only did all this invite retrospective reassessment of outbreaks; it invited reassessment of the assumptions one made on those frequent occasions where routes of transmission were unclear. Cholera was no longer exclusively fecal–oral. Food-borne, particularly crab-borne, outbreaks loomed larger, not because crabs were subject to sewage contamination, but because offshore crabs—both in their chitonous shells and in their guts—were an alternative host for vibrios. Traditionally, the assumption of asymptomatic carriers had been invoked when it proved impossible to identify all links in a presumed chain of transmission. Certainly, high rates of asymptomatic infection could be demonstrated; such "silent carriers" (aka ordinary, innocent-looking citizens) had assumed immense public-health importance. Writing at the height of the cold war, Pollitzer, who acknowledged a need to quarantine known contacts, was appalled at the measures some authorities proposed for treating all who could not prove otherwise as potentially guilty of smuggling of contraband vibrios. Given the alternative explanation of environmental reservoirs of cholera throughout the world, it could now be appreciated that "the role of long-term carriers of V. Cholerae O1 has . . . never been substantiated."

Initially focused on explaining the endemicity of cholera in Bengal, most of this new work was concerned with cholera as a marine organism: there has been no significant Pettenkoferian revival to explore it as a soil organism. And yet, as Glass and

Black pointed out in 1992, cholera was becoming endemic in interior African environments that would be expected to be "inhospitable to the marine vibrios."[9]

The new view had philosophical implications, equally for epistemology as for environmental ethics. The reason we had understood *Vibrio cholerae* so poorly was that we had been looking at it only through the very narrow lens of our own well-being. "Most cholera researchers fell in love with toxins and forgot that the vibrio ... producing them is an environmental organism and does not inhabit the intestinal tracts of humans simply to make them miserable," observed Stephen Richardson.[10]

A multi-perspectival approach would make clearer how cholera's occasional pathogenicity fit into the broader pattern of its life, and its pursuit of its needs. Each new standpoint altered subject and object. Our view of *Vibrio cholerae* was plain; what was its view of us? That required a perspectival reversal. Hitherto, cholera science had taken place outside the broader agendas of biology; success in responding to cholera had been mainly an engineering achievement: the building of safe water supplies. As we have seen, the very taxonomy of the vibrios had been infected by the agenda of human pathogencity, which now seemed an incidental (and even a transitory) property with no marked standing among the many elements of similarity and difference.

While that new perspectivalism left some emphasizing *Vibrio cholerae* as a "benign" member of a marine ecosystem (or an "innocuous estuarine-dweller"), it was quite clear that its suite of adaptations also made it a powerful pathogen. The quorum-sensing—changing its mode of operation based on the concentration of other members of its own or other species—that protected it at sea helped stimulate its virulence. Some strains could clump together to avoid extirpation by stomach acidity. Passage through the human intestine might itself turn on virulence. Writing of the complexity of toxin expression, Richardson observed that "it appears that human and bacterial systems are jockeying for an advantage," but then implored us to remember that "humans are just a temporary ecological niche for *V. cholerae*... we are really dealing with an estuarine-based bacterium trying to survive in two quite different worlds."[11] Like the hoods in *West Side Story*, cholera might simply be misunderstood.

All this involved repudiation of the truths of the laboratory: "a lazy life on an agar plate" was no good guide to how the microbe operated elsewhere, whether at sea or in the human gut.[12] The positing of a VBNC (viable but not culturable) state was particularly problematic. Here were bacteria defying the long-standing methodological maxim of bacteriology, in which viable implied culturable; one had only to supply the right medium. A mentality and set of techniques created for detecting microbes in clinical specimens, where they were concentrated, was ill-suited for drawing conclusions about marine environments where they were sparse. Yet divers in Chesapeake Bay or the Black Sea surfaced with greater levels of vibriocidal antibodies in their blood: evidently, they were acting as human culture plates. So, too, were residents of Bangladesh. There, "thousands of water samples might be analyzed without a single isolation of *V. cholerae* O1... At the same time, millions of people ingest water several times daily directly from these water sources, creating a much greater 'sampling' intensity..."[13]

But the makers of such qualifications did not follow them up in the same ways. Some saw the way forward as a more basic science: if the culture plate could not be trusted, better to go directly to the genome. Others held that *in vitro* methods were categorically inadequate, especially for making sense of immune response in humans. Antibody formation might sometimes be "in vivo-specific", a composite function of the presence of other gut flora, acidity, and "host-derived antibiotic factors." The longest-lasting immunity, it was noted, was that which came from acquiring the disease naturally. The lesson for some from a century and a quarter of vaccine development was that a live oral vaccine—the mode which came closest to getting cholera the natural way—worked best.

The language suggests how far things had evolved. Immunity, after all, had been (and is to most of us) a property we possess as living bodies; it is inherently *in vivo*. The claim in one review that the best correlate of antibacterial immunity was the quantity of vibriocidal antibody created by swallowing "wild" *Vibrio cholerae* will seem a truism, since we define our immunity as what happens if we accidentally swallow such stuff.

Modern cholera science is rife with hypotheses of what might be. The possibilities are more than speculations; cholera science has disclosed change and variability, and it has fostered humility: the vibrios had been underestimated, mischaracterized. Floating biofilm communities, colonization of crab shells and copepod innards, genetic exchanges with sinister phages—all fascinating biology, but had it anything to do with curing and preventing? In the century and a half during which cholera had been incurable and hard to prevent, there had been clear justification for a broad research front; now that it could be cured and prevented, what was to be the mission of cholera science? Just as all was revealed, revelation became irrelevant.

So secure is faith in the virtue of applied science that this critique is seldom voiced: yet one reads it between the lines, and in a few areas the tension is palpable. Since the early 1960s, wrote van Henyingen and Seal, cholera research had "passed into hands that had never dealt with the manifestations of the disease, even in experimental animals, let alone suffering humanity." They deplored the results: "it became more like everyday modern experimental biological science, more competitive and so less humane, less inspiring, less agreeable, less comradely."[14] The complaint was not new, nor newly warranted. The followers of Koch had wondered why latter-day Pettenkoferians kept amassing data on ground-water levels, when simply filtering the water would stop the scourge. But many of Koch's followers, too, had moved ever deeper into the laboratory. The only cholera they knew was in the cultures they exchanged.

If the theme of late-twentieth-century cholera science has been "complicate," that of cholera practice has been "simplify." "Simple and cheap" means more prevention and more cure. The exemplar is the move from IV to oral rehydration. Recognition that oral rehydrants would work if the salts were accompanied with some form of sugar brought with it an appreciation that staples like rice, prepared and administered by family members, could be mainstays of cholera therapy. Oral rehydrants would be distributed as solids, with instructions for mixing them up in local units—teaspoons, not cc's. In other cases, traditional remedies or preventives were shown to have had value after all, like lime juice, used in West Africa. Modest changes in tools, behavior, and diet (more acidic fish sauces) could prevent cholera. Small-scale water supplies could be made safe; narrow-necked vessels for household water storage lowered cholera rates enormously; filtration through sari-cloth removed cholera-bearing copepods in brackish waters.

Another prominent site of simplification was diagnosis. The distinctiveness of cholera was a central theme in its history, the source of the Asiatic stigma, and equally the occasion of magisterial achievements of epidemiology and bacteriology, which had proved the superiority of expert knowledge over lay. Following the frequent assertions of nineteenth-century authors that they, certainly, could distinguish Asiatic cholera from its feeble Western imitators (even if others could not), cholera's historians—Delaporte excepted—have privileged its uniqueness over its commonality with similar diseases. While the claims of these earlier authors now seem unduly confident, still we could take satisfaction that they had been vindicated by Koch. Thereafter, one could confirm clinical diagnosis by stool culture—and, since that might produce only a generic result, one could use antisera and other biochemical markers to pin down serogroup, biotype, serotype. Or, using more recondite means for reading the genome, one could test for virulence genes directly, or determine distinctiveness from other strains. But to what end?

In the case of diarrheal diseases, whether the disease was cholera or some other, the cure was the same and so probably were the means of prevention. The clinician gained little from diagnosing cholera. Mild cholera (most cases) would be indistinguishable from other diarrheas; more severe cases might be from other agents, including *E coli*. "For management of the individual patient...it is not necessary to know...The rehydration therapy is the same." The laboratory might be dangerous as well as superfluous. The early developers of modern rehydration therapy had insisted on calculating precisely how much water a victim had lost, fearing under- or over-hydration as a common cause of failure. It would soon be found that simple signs—pulse, eyes, skin turgor—were good enough. Diagnosis on the fly might be better. An experienced clinician would see complications that tests might not disclose. And speed was important: a "severely dehydrated patient may literally be within minutes of death unless hydration is instituted." The laboratory was for research but also for documentation. It might make no difference to clinicians if a disease were the real cholera, but it did to states, if they were to begrudge the resources needed to meet an epidemic.[15]

Typically, suspicion of cholera arose from indicators of epidemicity: only when the rate of severe diarrhea—in adults—suddenly rose did one think cholera might be present. Despite availability of quick biochemical means to detect its toxin directly, uniformity and familiarity often won out: the techniques used—microscopy, traditional stool culture, minimal serology—were comparatively primitive. With *Vibrio cholerae* confirmed, outside authorities would be notified. Since the cholera would not have been caught at the outset, retrospective diagnosis might be needed to track down an index case. Once enough cases had been cultured to confirm an epidemic, laboratory confirmation would again be suspended. It requires skilled labor and resources, both typically in short supply during an epidemic. However well warranted, such practices sacrifice precision; they reflect the considered judgment that culturing every sufferer adds little value.

The tension between clinic and laboratory allows cholera to be defined differently in different places. If a bacteriological definition seems the surer approach, in practice it will underrepresent: there must be a threshold of severity before anyone thinks to culture. Even then, the completeness of culturing will depend on facilities, skills, and budgets. The listing only of confirmed cases, coupled with underinvestment in the means to confirm, has been seen as a deliberate strategy to generate a low cholera count. More systematic culturing programs have targeted contacts of cholera victims, pilgrims to Mecca, or westbound travelers from Asia. Those programs identify large numbers of asymptomatic or subclinical cases. About 70 percent of those infected with *Vibrio cholerae* will be asymptomatic, a further 15–23 percent will have only mild cases. For epidemiological purposes these cases might be important; for clinical purposes, they would be false positives. In parts of Peru, symptomatic or aysmptomatic carriers would have included nearly everyone.

The alternative is to rely on a clinical definition. But not only do clinical definitions differ; they do not pretend that what is counted need be caused by *Vibrio cholerae* infection. Instead, they take us back before 1817, when "cholera" was a generic designation. Clinical factors in such designations include age, severity of dehydration, and epidemic incidence—that is, per capita diarrhea. But there are problems here too. Age-based definitions exclude children, on the grounds that childhood diarrhea has so many causes. Yet, where cholera is endemic, it is significantly a childhood disease. Adults have a relative immunity, having had the disease as children.

Acknowledging the diversity of reporting practices and the range of purposes for which the numbers may be used, the WHO cholera definition incorporates both cultural and clinical elements. Suspected cases are recognized clinically; once epidemic cholera has been confirmed by culture, cases may be counted if they have an "epidemiological linkage" to an outbreak.[16] That epidemical linkage argument presumes that cholera drives out other diarrheas: once it has been confirmed in a place, all diarrhea cases are counted as cholera. Yet, in a postflood diarrhea epidemic in Dhaka in 2004, the rate of cholera infection among hospitalized patients was only 22 percent. It is also assumed that a positive test for *Vibrio cholerae* in a person with diarrhea means that that person has cholera. Yet severe diarrhea may often be the result of more than one microbe. Such "mixed infections" would be reported as cholera if only *Vibrio cholerae* were being tested for.[17]

Following earlier international conventions, the WHO made cholera a notifiable disease in 1951, yet many countries flout its decree. As of 2005, Bangladesh, traditional homeland of cholera, did not report cases. The reasons for unwillingness to cooperate are familiar: nations fear loss of tourism, sanctions against trade, or other forms of hostile quarantine. The WHO thinks only 5–10 percent of cases of cholera (or, according to another source, only 1 percent) are reported to it. But even countries using its guidelines may not be using them consistently. Frustration with official statistics has led to a semi-formal network of epidemic reporting, overseen by the International Society of Infectious Diseases. And the vexed question "how much cholera is there really" is unanswerable so long as definitions are indefinite.

One may wonder if "cholera" has outlived its usefulness. It represents, after all, a medical system that gave us "hysteria" and "melancholia," diagnoses that not only do not illuminate but may do harm. The tracking of strains might still be important but for other purposes. "Acute watery diarrhea," which comprehends most cholera, is at least consistently clinical (though what counts as diarrhea is itself tricky). In the mid 1970s, the WHO did begin to recognize diarrhea as a generic problem, yet interest in cholera has persisted. Helping to sustain it was the inertia of research—first in its exemplary toxin, then in its fluctuating genome, more recently in its ecology. But it has also been kept in play by political, cultural, and economic factors.

CHOLERA: THE BIOGRAPHY

For starters, "cholera" has a grip on the public imagination that "acute watery diarrhoea" cannot match. That grip is disproportionate to its incidence. Even where cholera is endemic, other diarrheas are more common.[18] In 2005, 2,272 deaths from cholera were reported to the WHO. Yet about 1.6 million die annually of waterborne diseases. Roughly a third of these are probably from rotaviruses, which are not, like cholera, a household term. Yet the image of the single imported cholera case stepping off the airplane in some safe haven in the developed world (for example, somewhere in the United States) and triggering a diarrheal avalanche was hard to dismiss, notwithstanding the fact that the combination of prosperity, sanitary infrastructure, and elaborate public-health surveillance institutions made the prospect unlikely.

The most important area where diarrheal specificity made a difference was in vaccine development. Most means of prevention act against all forms of waterborne or fecal–oral diseases; vaccines act only against (certain strains of) *Vibrio cholerae*. Following decades of records of ambiguous effectiveness, the WHO removed cholera vaccination from its list of inoculations for international travelers in 1973. The verdict in the compendia that followed the Latin American outbreak in the early 1990s was unambiguous. Not only were cholera vaccines not a good idea; they were a bad one.

Beginning in the 1960s it had been demonstrated through cost–benefit studies that it was cheaper to treat cholera than to hope to eliminate it from endemic areas by vaccination. In terms of use of *public* funds, cure was better than prevention. Such calculations left out workdays lost to illness and the more dicey ethical problem that, in eschewing vaccines, one invited occurrence of avoidable cases of a potentially deadly illness. They did address another ethical issue: that reliance on a vaccine, partially effective for one relatively rare form of fecal–oral disease, would encourage risky behavior with regard to fecal–oral diseases generally. As Barua and Merson put it, "vaccination gives a false sense of security to those vaccinated, who consequently neglect more effective precautions, and rouse feelings of accomplishment and complacency among health authorities…Donations of vaccines may thus do more harm than good."[19] Exacerbating that false security was the brief effectiveness of cholera vaccines, rarely for more than a year. Finding that they remained subject to diarrheal diseases, vaccinees would lose faith in public health and modern medicine. By the 1990s it would become clear—at least to some—that *Vibrio cholerae*'s rapid adaptation made it unlikely that the vaccine problem could be solved in the long term.

Such considerations did nothing to slow vaccine development, however. Continued optimism reflected both the growing power to transform the cholera genome, and also the finding of a plausible context for use—not in mass vaccination campaigns but for pre-emptive strikes in refugee camps. Reliable sanitation and facilities for sufficient rehydration might be lacking in such places, while even limited vaccination lowered incidence, and hence opportunity for transmission. Vaccines were "a useful complement," and therefore worth developing.[20] Long-term cost effectiveness was not a major concern in the context of disaster relief. Vaccine advocates could point out, too, that, notwithstanding the effectiveness of ORT (oral rehydration therapy), there were parts of the world where cholera case mortality was more than 50 percent, a nineteenth-century figure, and that, notwithstanding decades of calls to invest in sanitary infrastructure to stay the scourge, water and sanitation lagged. This was particularly the case in parts of Africa, which was replacing Bangladesh as the center of world cholera. There, cholera was much more related to natural and political disaster.

And yet the results of vaccine development have continued to disappoint; vaccination was one of those areas of cholera science where what made sense in theory and worked *in vitro* and in animal trials, but often worked less well in human populations. What was needed, noted a 2005 reviewer, was a single-dose long-lasting cholera vaccine, effective against all serotypes, especially good for children, and cheap: "ironically, extensive research over the last two decades have yielded two tourist vaccines ... of short-term protection that are commercially available in some western countries." Vaccination remained expensive. It had not been cost-effective in the 1960s at $0.06 per vaccination. The vaccine used in the first Gulf War had cost $8; the tourist vaccine in use in 2005, about $30.[21] The market for tourist vaccines was not mainly a public-health market: tourists ran a very low risk of cholera.

That the rich, who could pay for vaccines, were not those at risk of cholera was a long-standing complaint. Even if the vaccine worked, would anyone pay? Tetanus persisted in Bangladesh, van Heyningen and Seal had pointed out. Vaccines were available; they were not used.

The assumption that vaccines would be used and paid for reflected faith in new institutions of cholera response. In the nineteenth century, cholera had been a problem of nations, then of communities, and, by the end, a delicate diplomatic matter within the community of nations. By the twenty-first century the most important cholera institutions were NGOs, blending into transnational quasi-governmental entities such as the WHO and the World Bank. These existed in creative tension with national governments, which often had to be cajoled, pressured, or bribed into cooperation. Colonialism was officially over; now a safe, busy, and profitable world rested on thoroughgoing accountability—to the international community, if not to the citizenry.

The WHO's rejection in 1973 of quarantine and similar measures of cholera control was part of a new globalism whose watchword was transparency. Cholera's spread could be stopped if it were caught early. Local lives could be saved too. But punitive means of prevention like restrictions on trade or human movement would only invite cholera denial. Hidden from the world's gaze, cholera would strengthen and spread. "Global" was to imply "universal," "disinterested," "optimal," and "technical":

> The battle can only be won if there is a *global political will* ... and an agreement not to impose restrictions on trade and traffic against countries affected by the disease. Such restrictions hinder frank notifications and *international cooperation* and, thus, prevent the handling of cholera control as a purely *technical* problem.[22]

The Americas were congratulated by the authors of a 1994 review: nations had

> kept borders open and have avoided futile epidemic control strategies such as quarantine, broad import restrictions, mass vaccination, or mass chemoprophylaxis. Open surveillance allowed the hemisphere to deliver the life-saving activities of treatment, surveillance, and education swiftly. Other countries that conceal their cholera are not likely to have the same success.[23]

But the one-worlders could not deliver what they preached. Faith in international bureaucracy was no match for fear. Cholera and rumors of cholera did hamper export trade and tourism in

Latin America in 1991; elsewhere cholera terror led sometimes to bizarre restrictions, as against ore importation. To admit cholera was to proclaim one's filthiness, squalor, corruption, and laziness, and to broadcast one's deadly power against others. All things being equal, if cholera were occurring, to deny it was entirely rational—and much cheaper—than to admit it.

Rational, perhaps, but impermissible. "Surveillance" coupled with the carrot of sanitation would both disclose needs (dangers) and direct the dollars where they were needed. Rather than rely on the stopgap of vaccination, the world should learn "another and far better way of preventing diarrheal diseases," lectured van Heyningen and Seal: "not ingesting the faeces of diarrhea patients." This deadly coprophagy had been eliminated in the West; the same must now happen everywhere.

Surely few drank diarrheal discharges voluntarily; the dark sarcasm reflects frustration that obvious needs were not being met. "Such provision in the diarrhoea-endemic countries of the world is for the present only a distant dream," they admitted in these early years of the UN's Water and Sanitation Decade, adding that "perhaps the politicians whose duty it is to realize that dream should not be diverted from that duty by taking the easy but useless way out of flying in packages of vaccine, whether useless or not, in times of epidemic crisis."[24]

Cholera remained "a metaphor for underdevelopment," just as it had been almost two centuries earlier.[25] A golden age of world sanitation has been a central theme throughout the postwar era of "development." To many, sanitation still seems a way beyond cycles of poverty and disease, perhaps the only way. Whether realistic prospect or only the most recent version of a utopian technical millennium, faith in sanitary infrastructure has been compelling enough to inspire heroic effort and even to loosen purse strings. International campaigns were repeatedly launched with great fanfare but mixed results: the Water and Sanitation decade of the 1980s achieved much, but barely kept up with population growth. At the beginning of the twenty-first century, more than a billion lack safe water; more than double that, approaching a third of the world's population, lack adequate sanitation. The resurgence of interest in vaccination reflects the perceived failure of the Water and Sanitation Decade. Will the Millennium Goals do better? Certainly there are grounds for cynicism.

Again, or still, cholera has created moral problems as well as reflecting them. The waterworks that were to be public often turned out to be partial and private. The piped water and sewers of upscale hotels or gated communities amplified social distance when compared with the flying toilets of Kibera, the plastic bags used for defecation and then hurled into lanes or ditches. Here, enacted in pipe, were new forms of social division and new questions of inequality.

Supposedly, the clarion call of cholera was to redress that inequality. The 1994 announcement by Tauxe et al. that "the future of epidemic cholera will be defined by the course of modern periurban poverty" was a warning.[26] As in the nineteenth century, the menace of the contagious poor might be the only thing that could shift the apathetic rich. The industrialized world, too, must be reminded that it was not "entirely secure." In that light, the offshore presence of autochthonous *Vibrio cholerae* in the US gulf coast and in Australian rivers took on a special significance. Only give it rein, and the complacent developed world too would revert to the horrid nineteenth century. Cholera, Gangarosa and Tauxe observed, provided "leverage to persuade decision makers who control purse strings to reorder priorities and make the commitment of resources needed to correct the root problems." Some went so far as to claim that cholera could be a "net benefit to humanity by calling attention to deficiencies in basic systems and services that need to be corrected." There was to be a " 'Sanitary Reform' revolution in each affected country," just as had happened in Europe and the United States a century earlier.[27]

Most historians do not agree that cholera was the great stimulus. Rather, those wanting waterworks or sewers found in the threat of cholera epidemics good public reason for getting others to pay for them. But no matter. If the prospect of cholera—a different matter from its incidence—helps us talk our way into providing public goods, it will be a friend.

What precisely a modern sanitary revolution would look like was problematic. Two decades ago, most would have seen the sanitary apotheosis as the piped city, a high-pressure hydraulic achievement of sparkling water and powerful flush. More recently, many have recognized that the money will go further with more modest appliances. Perhaps it must do so, for someone has to pay. Diarrheal disease might well be an important determinant of poverty, but, if poverty were the limiting factor, the attempt to bootstrap out of it by incurring massive debt—an approach tried repeatedly during the development era—might be self-defeating.

Questions about how to prevent cholera were part of broader criticisms of an emulation model of development. Recognizing that pipe dreams were exactly that, many sought means of cholera prevention that circumvented failing states and corrupt officials. For all sorts of reasons—ethical, social, cultural, geographic, and environmental—it might be that other parts of the world could not and should not follow the path of the USA and

Europe. But they might not need to. Perhaps cholera prevention did not require piped water to all. Billions of people *did* live in shanty towns, however much we might deplore that. Making the slums healthy may seem to approach oxymoron, but it could be done. Leaving aside vaccination, seen as an admission of inevitable failure, what then were the minimal requirements for a cholera-free society?

And yet this was an ambivalent inquiry. Pushed hard, the celebrations of simplicity rarely lent themselves to simple moral tales. That there were good low-tech means of dealing with cholera did not mean there might not be better high-tech ones. Cheap remedies might be well suited to poverty, but, in accepting them, one was acquiescing in that poverty. At some point realistic meeting of minimum needs crossed into a denial of aspiration to common standards.

One area of conflict was antibiotics. Rehydration alone was usually sufficient to cure cholera, but the vibrio was susceptible to antibiotics. In the 1960s, antibiotics had seemed an obvious complement to rehydration (then done mainly through IV). By shortening the dangerous stage of diarrhea, it would allow hospitals to serve more people. The result of this practice, evolution of antibiotic-resistant strains, led to its general abandonment. But antibiotics still helped, were sometimes used, and could be bought. The old view of tetracycline as "drug of choice for the treatment of cholera, whenever possible" still surfaces.[28] And did many victims really want the voluntary simplicity of antibiotic-free treatment?

There were other loci of ambivalence. All very well that sari cloth could filter copepods, but, used to clean babies' bottoms, it was also a means of transmission. Very nice that rice, a staple in many of the world's cholera centers, could complement ORT;

but contaminated leftover rice (or, in Africa, millet), along with many other food leftovers in places without refrigeration, was an excellent means of cholera transmission.

Water itself was a site of conflict. For decades, the focus on cholera control had been modern waterworks. The very decades during which it was becoming clear that waterworks could not be provided everywhere also marked a shift from the view of cholera as primarily a waterborne disease. Episodes like Hamburg in 1892, long emblematic in cholera's history, were increasingly looked upon as atypical. Modern epidemiologists were finding that much cholera was food-borne, or spread by many means in domestic and local settings. But how to interpret? Partisans of Snow or Koch might insist that cholera was rare in the developed world *because* cities were protected by sound mains, well-monitored filters, chlorine, and waste-water treatment. Yet others would point to growing evidence that improving water supplies did not necessarily bring down cholera levels.

Drawing on experience of under-maintained waterworks in developing countries, many experts were warning that they could not be trusted. "Large urban water systems may function as efficient distributors of contaminated water," noted commentators on the Latin American epidemic. Intermittency of service, producing temporary periods of low pressure, might allow ingress of sewage into poorly maintained pipes. Often, fecal coliform numbers rose with distance from the waterworks. Water storage might cause problems. In such conditions even central chlorination was unreliable. It required electricity for pumps, and a supply of chlorine. Neither could be guaranteed.[29]

This was no new truth, but it was taking on a new valence. Often it was less a call for better infrastructure and expert oversight than a fundamental challenge to public infrastructural solutions. On matters of water safety, one was on one's own. As with vaccination, some worried that efforts to control cholera through centralized water supplies fed a false security. "It is a peculiar irony of modern life in the developing world that large and poorly maintained water systems may be more hazardous than traditional water sources if the community believes that water is safe just because it comes from a pipe."[30] Dashed hopes would undercut confidence in science and public health. For, as in the nineteenth century, the most serious threat cholera posed was not death, but public order: "it is relatively easy to begin educating a population that water from a river or stream is unsafe and needs further treatment; it can be *politically explosive* to tell them that municipal water at the tap is not to be trusted."[31]

That the solution to the problem of inadequate public services was to make them better no longer seemed credible. But relying on each to be the judge of his or her own water needs and uses was hardly better. Scarcity of water led to its storage and reuse and to failure to wash bodies and things well or frequently. However high fecal coliforms might be in mains water, they were often higher in water in household storage. Retail water vending—long looked on as a mark of the bad old days—was not a good solution; bottled water had been the mode of transmission of a Portuguese outbreak in 1974. Boiling was an old standby, but not a realistic one because of high fuel costs, or always an effective one, since boiled water might be recontaminated during storage. The great technical solution of the 1990s, then, was the narrow-necked jar.

Ironically, then, just as it was becoming plain that all could not aspire to Western water and sanitation, it was being made clear, under the rubric of realistic solutions, that those mod cons were not so great after all. You cannot have it; but you do not really need it; you would not have liked it; probably you do not really want it.

In any case, water had been displaced from its long-standing role as primary cholera medium. No other single means of transmission took its place. Much cholera was being seen in some way as food-borne. Foods might account both for primary transmission of the pathogen into the human community, and, through food handling, distribution, and domestic storage practices, for its extension. Handwashing became a decisive cholera preventive and there was renewed interest in fly-borne transmission.

But many authorities were warning against expectation of a single route of transmission. In the midst of an outbreak, the vibrio might be coming by many routes to constitute an inoculum of critical mass. Victims' accounts of how they thought they had gotten the disease were not to be trusted. Underwriting this emerging view were both the growing pile of detections of *Vibrio cholerae* in ever more media and the new techniques of risk-factor epidemiology. Case-matching could reveal dimensions in which stricken and unstricken differed, sometimes suggesting unappreciated modes of transmission. While they would not dethrone John Snow, authors did take issue with his inferences. If *Vibrio cholerae* were found in the water of those getting cholera, it did not follow that the former was the cause of the latter: "simply demonstrating *V. cholerae* in a suspected water source does not by itself prove that the water was the source of infection for people; it may be a coincidental finding, occurring because persons infected from another source also happen to contaminate the water."[32]

The relocation of the central front of cholera control from expert management of a municipal waterworks to household and community practices marks a return to what has been called the "moral" stage of public health. States were giving cholera back to individuals, at the same time as making it too complicated for rational response. As in the 1830s, cholera is to be prevented by the discipline of ordinary persons taking the harder not the easier way. Risk-factor epidemiology proved a tool of remarkable fertility for generating long lists of ways to avoid cholera. Important to know, for example, that "persons who smoked cannabis more than twice a week were at increased risk of developing diarrhea following ingestion of V. *cholerae* O1 compared with persons who did not smoke cannabis or who smoked cannabis less frequently." The result, note the authors, may have implications for the Ganges delta, "where cannabis use is common among certain segments of the population."[33] (Henceforth one will confine one's doping to once weekly, all the while regretting not having been able to participate in the trials that established this worthy result.) Here the culprit was a lowering of stomach acid, which had re-emerged as the front line of cholera defense. By contrast, beer-drinkers were relatively safe.

Cholera, it seems, can be controlled only by disciplining the poor. The irony is staggering. Recognizing the futility of sermons, which had so often been looked upon as hypocrisy and received with contempt, to alter cholera-causing behaviors, the sanitarians of the 1840s had sought a Benthamite solution. Do not appeal to some presumed conscience, they say; simply adjust structures to alter the vector sum of pains and pleasures to obtain the desired mass behavior. With plentiful, high pressure, high-quality water laid on in the home, there was no need to preach cleanliness. Excrement would vanish; clothes, bodies, and dishes would be washed because the pleasures of water and soap, and of health and cleanliness, so clearly outweighed the work of achieving them. Dwellings, with the people in them, became self-cleaning machines: water and sewerage did all that was asked because they operated automatically.

This new burden of cholera prevention, by contrast, is often inconvenient, laborious, and expensive. Prevention is a zero-sum game, precisely the condition the sanitarians hoped to avoid. One trades some safety for cheapness and convenience. In such conditions, the work of the lowest of the low-tech interventions, that of the health educator, often collapses into didacticism. One hopes simply to shift the trade-off point more toward the pole of disease avoidance.

Cholera prevention authorities struggled to avoid suggesting that they were requiring cultures to change. In the postcolonial environment, there was great concern that development be freely chosen. By the 1990s, a widespread frustration with lodging that autonomy in states had evolved; all too often these were failed states; sometimes they had failed more than once. Instead, the site of hygienic change was to be the "community," an imagined utopia that would effect the marriage of the true democracy of the New England town meeting with the newest cholera prevention measures. The health educator's role was that of facilitator, to help community members reach through their own processes of decision-making precisely the conclusion the educator would have them reach. The community itself would institute the necessary cholera-preventing changes. This strategy required tact, patience, the (apparent) devolution of power from expert to lay person, and, sometimes, willingness to back community decisions even if these were not technically ideal.

Writing in the more authoritarian 1950s, when colonies still existed, Pollitzer had seen no need for such delicacy. He wrote of the role of health "propaganda" in cholera control at a time when "propaganda" had not yet become a dirty word. Modern cholera writers had greater difficulty. A balance had to be struck between science and community process, but they dithered about where to strike it. Writing on "The prevention and Control of Cholera," Barua and Merson stressed that "communication should go beyond attempts to educate by didactic methods and use a two-way approach to involve and motivate people." But any listening, evidently, was instrumental: (pretend to) listen to get others to do what they need to do.[34]

The meanings that would be given to cholera were important, and had to be managed. This spin-doctoring was more than mere transparency. Again the problem was little different from what it had been in the 1830s. The antidote to "exaggerated rumors" was "carefully designed messages." These "correct messages" were to be "based on the beliefs and practices of the people." British cholera policy in late-nineteenth-century India had made a point of not interfering with religious practices— albeit for cynical reasons of maintaining political stability while avoiding expense. By the 1990s religious practices were seen as fungible, and religious and community leaders useful only to the degree that they could be led. On the fraught question of disposal of the dead, Barua and Merson insisted that "funerals of persons dying from cholera should take place quickly, near the place of death; efforts should be made to restrict funeral gatherings, ritual washing and touching of the dead, and especially feasting, by intensive health education or by legislation."[35]

That we have, in many respects, returned to recognize problems that were central at earlier stages of cholera's history, begun to take seriously questions, complexity, and forms of evidence that were neglected for long periods, begun to give more attention to minimal changes that will lessen diarrhea incidence over the vast and visionary transformations that were to prevent it, may be all to the good. More than at any other time in its history, the response to cholera seems realistic.

But another way to view that transformation is as the reconstitution of cholera as simply a technical problem. We saw cholera become laden with meaning in the early nineteenth century— linked not only to providence and progress, but to liberal norms of citizenship and social justice, and to emerging institutions of democracy. What is happening now is an attempt to excise meaning. Cholera can be managed much more effectively, it is argued, if we get rid of the extraneous issues.

One of these is poverty. Barua and Merson observe that "the problem of cholera will ultimately be solved only when water supplies, sanitation and hygienic practices attain such a level that fecal–oral transmission of *V. cholerae* O1 becomes an improbable event" and that "this cannot happen without a marked amelioration of social and economic conditions in the developing world." They are not in fact declaring that such amelioration is imperative, but rather recognizing the need for pragmatic and immediate techniques to circumvent the absence of structural reform.[36]

Yet quite what would constitute a technical solution for a phenomenon which, as the geographer Andrew Collins sums it up, is subject to the "changing microecology of *V. cholerae*, vulnerability of people through exposure to health risks, resistance to infection through immunity and/or nutrition status, and environmental, socio-economic, and behavioral changes" is not at all clear.[37]

In fact there is no such thing as an exclusively technical solution. We cannot get rid of meaning, nor should we want to. Cholera will remain political and ethical. We should not apologize for it being a moral matter. Viewing, and not without good grounds, the nineteenth-century sanitary revolution as a democratic achievement, Tauxe et al. predict that "epidemic cholera is likely to be less and less tolerable in the growing democracies of Latin America."[38] And yet it is not at all clear whether democracies can be trusted to prioritize cholera, and it seems unlikely that they will do so unless it can be made to mean something very important to them.

It may be argued that campaigns against diarrheal diseases are inherently campaigns for justice and equality. Thus: the sources of diarrheal disease—not just cholera—are so widespread that to acquiesce to its endemic presence in any population is to put at risk every population, including wealthy populations that think they may build enough walls to keep it away. This is precisely the argument of the *Cholera Chaunt*. Such arguments are often implicit in what might be called a liberal perspective toward cholera, which is, broadly speaking, the one within which I write. Within such a framework, the finding of strains of *Vibrio cholerae* existing independently off the US coast binds Americans more closely to Bangladeshis or Africans, for whom that potential is often reality. Such a "there but for the grace of God go I" sensibility often lies at the core of ethical defenses of democracy.

What will be the contexts of that sense of diarrheal universality in the future? I suggest two. One is climate change. Much interest in the climatic determinants of cholera reflects recognition that, as sea levels and sea surface temperatures rise, the niche of *Vibrio cholerae* will expand. With new regions exposed directly, cholera will again be a world problem. Second is over-population. Here the links are both optimistic and pessimistic. Many researchers have already treated the problem of diarrheal disease, particularly among infants, in terms of the demographic transition. High infant death rates reflect (in part) population density, but they also contribute to cycles of poverty and are seen to block the aspirations of women, which are to be the trigger of reduced birth rates and eventual population stability. On the other side, many contemporary outbreaks of diarrheal disease are themselves consequences of ethnic rivalries, situations where different groups are trying to access the same resources.

Cholera will not disappear nor cease to mean. A great challenge will be to respond to the meanings it is given.

GLOSSARY

BIOTYPE, SEROGROUP, and **SEROTYPE** are terms that arose in the twentieth century to distinguish varieties of cholera vibrio: the **biotypes**, classical and eltor, were distinguished by behavior in culture and clinical, and epidemiological factors; **serogroups** and **serotypes** were classifications based on characteristic sets of cell surface antigens, molecules that triggered immune system responses

CHOLERA MORBUS a traditional term at the beginning of the nineteenth century for a malign form of humoral readjustment resulting in a dangerous discharge of bile

CHOLERA NOSTRAS after 1830, *cholera morbus* would evolve into *cholera nostras*, to distinguish a sporadic and relatively mild disease from the pandemic disease that was thought to come from India

COMMA BACILLUS Robert Koch's term for the cholera-causing microbe he isolated in 1883–4; the modern term is *Vibrio cholerae*

CONTAGIONISM, CONTINGENT CONTAGIONISM a group of theories of disease causation, attributing diseases (both specific disease entities or pathological influences more broadly) to something transmitted from sufferer (or later, carrier) to new victim; **contingent contagionism** refers to theories in which media of transmission between sufferer and victim are important factors;

anticontagionism is sometimes equated with miasmatism, but the term can and does comprehend a much broader range of causal factors, ranging from the social to the geophysical

ENDEMIC refers to the ongoing or sporadic incidence of a disease within a particular location; cholera was traditionally considered endemic to Bengal; it periodically became pandemic as it spread from there to the rest of the world

ENDOTOXIN, EXOTOXIN an **endotoxin** produces its pathological effects as the bacterial cell is destroyed; an **exotoxin** is released by a bacterium under certain conditions; while cholera has endotoxic effects, its major action is now known to be due to an exotoxin, usually labeled Ctx

EPIDEMIC a local transitory flare-up of a disease, which may be part of a global pandemic

FECAL–ORAL a disease transmitted by ingestion of an agent excreted in the feces of a sufferer or carrier; cholera's status as a fecal–oral disease is attributed to John Snow, who recognized a variety of means by which fecal matter might be ingested, but saw contaminated water as the main means of epidemic extension; modern science sees cholera as often but not always fecal–oral

GASTROENTERITIS a clinical condition of diarrhea and vomiting, which may be more or less severe; both early in its history and more recently, cholera has not always been distinguished from other severe gastroenteritis

HUMORAL THEORIES theories of pathology, prominent in antiquity and in the early modern period, and still influential in the early nineteenth century, that interpret illness in terms of imbalances among the body's primary fluids; in Western Europe, the most familiar of these theorized four primary fluids: blood, phlegm, yellow bile, and black bile; Indian and Chinese medical systems were also broadly humoral

ILEUM   the section of the small intestine where the toxic effects of the cholera vibrio are most marked, in causing the passing of water across the intestinal wall

MIASMATISM   a group of theories of disease causation, attributing many diseases to an infection from an invisible, and possibly otherwise undetectable, emanation from rotting organic matter—swamps, sewers, or filthy cities; miasmatic theories were prominent well into the middle of the nineteenth century

ORAL REHYDRATION THERAPY (ORT)   the main modern means of treatment of cholera and other forms of gastro-enteritis that produce serious dehydration; though tried sporadically over the centuries, rehydration (often intravenously or by injection beneath the skin) became the standard after 1960 as it was recognized what kinds of chemical balances might need to be re-established in returning a victim to health

PANDEMIC   a disease outbreak occurring over a wide geographic area and affecting an exceptionally high proportion of the population; in the cholera literature the term refers to periodic waves of the disease that cover much of the world; cholera was traditionally considered **endemic** to Bengal; it periodically became pandemic as it spread from there to the rest of the world

PHAGE a virus capable of infecting a bacterium, altering its viability or its genetic makeup; in cholera, phages have been important as prophylactic agents, and also for tracing patterns of cholera transmission; the action of phages also helps to account for cholera's toxicity

PLEOMORPHISM the phenomena of morphological and other changes in bacteria due to changed environmental conditions; for much of the twentieth century pleomorphic considerations challenged notions of the stability of bacterial species

POSITIVISM a philosophy of scientific practice emphasizing the avoidance of speculative mechanisms and abstractions in favor of correlations among measurable facts; that practice, if not the philosophy, is reflected in the contemporary focus on identifying risk factors

RECRUDESCENCE the view that a new outbreak in a region reflects the re-emergence or revivification of microbes that have been existing in the local environment rather than a new importation of the disease from another place

VIBRIO in general, a curved, rod-shaped bacterium, now a genus of bacteria; following Filipo Pacini, the agent of cholera is now known as *Vibrio cholerae*; because cholera is the most interesting of the genus, other vibrios are sometimes collectively labeled NCV, or non-cholera vibrios; among cholera vibrios, serotypes O1 and O139 are capable of producing epidemic disease; before the discovery of O139 in the early 1990s, non-pathogenic varieties of *Vibrio cholerae* were known collectively as non-O1

ZYMOTIC common as a descriptor of the mode of pathological action of a variety of diseases now regarded as infectious or contagious; the term uses the metaphor of fermentation to understand the destructive effect that the introduction of a minute amount of decomposing matter might have on the body's tissues and fluids; historically, zymotic explanations mediated between environmental and miasmatic explanations of disease and contagionist germ theoretic explanations

NOTES

Prologue

1. Ira Klein, "Imperialism, Ecology, and Disease," *Indian Economic and Social History Journal*, 31/4 (1994), 491–518, at 429.

2. The authority is R. Pollitzer, "History of Cholera," *Bulletin of the WHO*, 10 (1954), 421–61, at 422ff; cf Patrice Bourdelais and Jean-Yves Raulot, *Une peur bleue: Histoire du choléra en France, 1832–1854* (Paris, 1987), 13–45.

3. Pierre Dorolle, 'International Surveillance of Cholera', in Dhiman Barua and William Burrows (eds), *Cholera* (Philadelphia, 1974), 427–33, at 429.

4. Norman Howard-Jones, "Choleranomalies: The Unhistory of Medicine as Exemplified by Cholera," *Perspectives in Biology and Medicine*, 15 (1972), 422–33, at 422.

5. Roderick McGrew, "The First Cholera Epidemic and Social History," *Bulletin of the History of Medicine*, 34 (1960), 61–73, at 64.

6. Louis Chevalier, "Introduction générale," in Louis Chevalier (ed.), *Le Choléra: La Première Épidémie due XIXe siècle* (La Roche-sur-Yon, 1958), iii–xvii; Roderick McGrew, "The First Cholera Epidemic and Social History," *Bulletin of the History of Medicine*, 34 (1960), 61–73; Asa Briggs, "Cholera and Society," *Past and Present*, 119 (1961), 76–96; Charles Rosenberg, *The Cholera Years: The United States in 1832, 1849, and 1866* (Chicago, 1962); id., "Cholera in Nineteenth Century Europe: A Tool for Social and Economic Analysis," *Comparative Studies in Society and History*, 8 (1966), 452–63.

7. Rosenberg, *The Cholera Years*, 4.

8. McGrew, "The First Cholera Epidemic," 71.

Chapter 1

1. Robert James, *Medicinal Dictionary* (3 vols; London, 1743–5), s.v. "Cholera."

2. John Heysham, *Observations on the Bills of Mortality, in Carlisle, for the Year MDCCLXXXIII* (Carlisle, 1784), 4.

3. John Macpherson, *Annals of Cholera from the Earliest Period to the Year 1817* (2nd edn, London, 1884), 7–11.

4. [R. Hooper], *A Compendious Medical Dictionary* (London, 1798), s.v. "Cholera."

5. James, "Cholera."

6. Alfred Stillé, *Cholera: Its Origin, History, Causation, Symptoms, Lesions, Prevention, and Treatment* (Philadelphia, 1885), 145.

7. John Murray, *Observations on the Pathology and Treatment of Cholera* (New York, 1874), 25; F. Bisset Hawkins, *History of the Spasmodic Cholera of Russia; Including a Copious Account of the Disease which has Prevailed in India, and which has Travelled, under that Name, from Asia into Europe* (London, 1831), 97; Ira Klein, "Cholera: Theory and Treatment in Nineteenth Century India," *Journal of Indian History* (1980), 35–51, at 40.

8. Archibald Pitcairn, *The Philosophical and Mathematical Elements of Physick* (2 vols, 2nd edn, London, 1745), ii. 249–50.

9. James Lind, *An Essay on Diseases Incidental to Europeans in Hot Climates* (2nd edn, London, 1771), 275.

10. Benjamin Rush, *Medical Inquiries and Observations* (London, 1794), 131–2, 135.

11. Macpherson, *Annals*, 42–77; Raoul Henri Scoutetten, *A Medical and Topographical History of the Cholera Morbus, Including the Mode of Prevention and Treatment*, trans. A. Sidney Doane (Boston, 1832), 45; Hawkins, *Spasmodic Cholera of Russia*, 127.

12. James Kennedy, *The History of the Contagious Cholera, with Facts Explanatory of its Origin and Laws, and a Rational Method of Cure* (2nd edn, London, 1832), 26–34.

13. Hardin Weatherford, *A Treatise on Cholera, with the Causes, Symptoms, Mode of Prevention and Cure, on a New and Successful Plan* (Louisville, 1833), 47.

14. Scoutetten, *Medical and Topographical History*, 32, 36.

15. Whitelaw Ainslie, *Observations on the Cholera Morbus of India: A Letter Addressed to the Honourable Court of Directors of the East-India Company* (London, 1825), 78–9.

16. Macpherson, *Annals*, 28; cf Julius Jolly, *Indian Medicine*, trans. with notes by C. G. Kashikar (3rd edn, New Delhi, 1994), 90–2.

17. N. Charles Macnamara, *A History of Asiatic Cholera* (London, 1876), pp. vii–ix.

18. Macpherson, *Annals*, 42, 14; cf N. Howard-Jones, "Choleranomalies: The Unhistory of Medicine as Exemplified by Cholera," *Perspectives in Biology and Medicine*, 15 (1972), 422–33, at 428.

19. Macpherson, *Annals*, 42–95; James Bontius, *An Account of the Diseases, Natural History, and Medicines, of the East Indies. To which are Added Annotations by a Physician* (London, 1769), 26–9; R. H. Scoutetten, *Histoire Chronologique Topographique et Étymologique du Choléra depuis la Haute Antiquité jusqu'a son Invasion en France en 1832* (Paris, 1869), 17.

20. *The Cholera Bulletin* [New York], Aug. 20, 1832.

21. Rush, *Medical Inquiries*, 132; Macpherson, *Annals*, 75, 207–23; Stillé, *Cholera*, 107–12; S. N. De, *Cholera: Its Pathology and Pathogenesis* (Edinburgh, 1961), 31–2.

22. Murray, *Observations*, 23; Ainslie, *Cholera*, 52–3; Myron M. Levine and Nathaniel F. Pierce, "Immunity and Vaccine Development," in Dhiman Barua and William Burrows (eds), *Cholera* (Philadelphia, 1974), 285–327, at 287; Eric S. Krukonis and Victor J. DiRita, "From Motility to Virulence: Sensing and Responding to Environmental Signals in *Vibrio Cholerae*," *Current Opinion in Microbiology*, 6 (2003), 186–90, at 187.

23. Macnamara, *History*, v, 28–33.

24. Macnamara, *History*, 35–6; Macpherson, *Annals*, 115–17, 159.

25. Joseph Fayrer, *The Natural History and Epidemiology of Cholera* (London, 1888), 16; cf Kennedy, *Contagious Cholera*, ch. 1.

26. R. Pollitzer, "Cholera Studies: 1. History of the Disease," *Bulletin of the World Health Organization*, 10 (1954), 421–61, at 427.

27. August Hirsch, *Handbook of Historical and Geographical Pathology. Vol. 1. Acute Infective Diseases* (London, 1883), 394–437.

28. Vijay Prashad, "Native Dirt/Imperial Ordure: The Cholera of 1832 and the Morbid Resolutions of Modernity," *Journal of Historical Sociology* (1994), 243–60 at 247.

29. Macpherson, *Annals*, 90–8.

Chapter 2

1. Charles E. Rosenberg, *The Cholera Years: The United States in 1832, 1849, and 1866* (Chicago, 1962), 42.

2. David Arnold, "Cholera and Colonialism in British India," *Past and Present*, 113 (1986), 118–51; Charles Briggs and Clara Mantini-Briggs, *Stories in the Time of Cholera: Racial Profiling during a Medical Nightmare* (Berkeley and Los Angeles, 2003).

3. Briggs and Mantini-Briggs, *Stories*, 26, 296–7.

4. Briggs and Martini-Briggs, *Stories*, 33.

5. James Annesley, *Sketches of the Most Prominent Diseases of India; Comprising a Treatise on the Epidemic Cholera of the East; Statistical and Topographical Reports of the Diseases of the Different Divisions of the Army under the Madras Presidency* ... (2nd edn, London, 1829).

6. F. Bisset Hawkins, *History of the Spasmodic Cholera of Russia; Including a Copious Account of the Disease which has Prevailed in India, and which has Travelled, under that Name, from Asia into Europe* (London, 1831) 170.

7. Reginald Orton, *An Essay on the Epidemic Cholera of India* (2nd edn, London, 1831), 434–7, 451–4.

8. James Christie, *Cholera Epidemics in East Africa* (London, 1876), 274–5, 301.

NOTES TO PP. 62–70

9. Christie, *Cholera Epidemics in East Africa*, 289–96.

10. Hawkins, *Spasmodic Cholera of Russia*, 95–6, 123, emphasis in original.

11. Orton, *Epidemic Cholera*, 455 n.; Hawkins, *Spasmodic Cholera of Russia*, 179; cf R. H. Scoutetten, *A Medical and Topographical History of the Cholera Morbus, Including the Mode of Prevention and Treatment*, trans. A. Sidney Doane (Boston, 1832), 57.

12. Arnold, "Cholera," 120–2.

13. Scoutetten, *Medical and Topographical History*, 10–16.

14. R. Nelson, *Asiatic Cholera: Its Origin and Spread in Asia, Africa, and Europe, Introduction into America through Canada; Remote and Proximate Causes, Symptoms and Pathology, and the Various Modes of Treatment Analyzed* (New York, 1866), 143.

15. R. H. Scoutetten, *Histoire Chronologique Topographique et Étymologique du Choléra depuis la Haute Antiquité jusqu'a son Invasion en France en 1832* (Paris, 1869), 18–19.

16. John Macpherson, *Annals of Cholera from the Earliest Period to the Year 1817* (2nd edn, London, 1884), 155.

17. Orton, *Epidemic Cholera*, 436–7.

18. Orton, *Epidemic Cholera*, 59–60.

19. Hawkins, *Spasmodic Cholera of Russia*, 11–12.

20. E. O. Shakespeare, *Report on the Cholera in Europe and India* (Washington, 1890), 194.

21. Quoted in John Austin, *Cholera Morbus: A Short and Faithful Account of the History, Progress, Causes, Symptoms, and Treatment of the Indian and Russian Cholera, Taken from Authentic Sources, with Cases as Related by Practitioners in India* (London, 1831), 43–4.

22. Quoted in Orton, *Epidemic Cholera*, 456; emphasis added.

23. Michael Roth, "The Western Cholera Trail: Studies in the Urban Response to Epidemic Disease in the Trans-Mississippi West, 1848–1850" (PhD dissertation, Santa Barbara, 1993), 208; Annesley, quoted in Hawkins, *Spasmodic Cholera of Russia*, 11.

311

24. Shakespeare, *Report on the Cholera in Europe and India*, 113.

25. Hawkins, *Spasmodic Cholera of Russia*, 124, 179; Austin, *Cholera Morbus*, 6; Scoutetten, *Medical and Topographical History*, 63.

26. Orton, *Epidemic Cholera*, 146.

27. Austin, *Cholera Morbus*, 6.

28. Rosenberg, *The Cholera Years*, 16.

29. Nelson, *Asiatic Cholera*, 58–60; Shakespeare, *Report on the Cholera in Europe and India*, 361.

30. Hawkins, *Spasmodic Cholera of Russia*, 40; Ira Klein, "Imperialism, Ecology, and Disease," *Indian Economic and Social History Journal*, 31/4 (1994), 491–518, at 504; David Arnold, *Colonizing the Body: State Medicine and Epidemic Disease in Nineteenth-Century India* (Berkeley and Los Angeles, 1993), 184.

31. Sir B. Baker, quoted in Christie, *Cholera Epidemics in East Africa*, 66, 92.

32. Christie, *Cholera Epidemics in East Africa*, 88–92; Klein, "Imperialism," 503.

33. Cyrus Hamlin, *Among the Turks* (New York, 1877), 313–14.

34. Hamlin, *Among the Turks*, 305–12.

35. Hamlin, *Among the Turks*, 305–7.

36. Hamlin, *Among the Turks*, 307.

37. James Kennedy, *The History of the Contagious Cholera, with Facts Explanatory of its Origin and Laws, and a Rational Method of Cure* (2nd edn, London, 1832), 23.

38. Scoutetten, *Medical and Topographical History*, 22, 28, 52–5.

39. Quoted in Rosenberg, *The Cholera Years*, 44; see also 121.

40. François Delaporte. *Disease and Civilisation, the Cholera in Paris, 1832*, trans. A. Goldhammer (Cambridge, MA, 1986), 34–52.

41. Quoted in Shakespeare, *Report on the Cholera in Europe and India*, 137.

42. Frank Snowden, *Naples in the Time of Cholera, 1884–1911* (Cambridge, 1995), 241.

43. Orton, *Epidemic Cholera*, 133–44.

44. Nelson, *Asiatic Cholera*, 75–7, 160–4.

45. Rosenberg, *The Cholera Years*, 2 n.

46. Scoutetten, *Medical and Topographical History*, 56; "A Fact for Non-Contagionists," *Cholera Bulletin*, 8, July, 23 1832, 60.

47. Shakespeare, *Report on the Cholera in Europe and India*, 127.

48. "First Sermon on the Cholera," in Charles Kingsley, *Sermons on National Subjects* (London, 1890), 137, 139, 142; Pamela Gilbert, *Cholera and Nation: Doctoring the Social Body in Victorian England* (Albany, NY, 2008), 40.

49. Kingsley, "Second Sermon" and "Third Sermon," in *Sermons*, 144–52, 153–63, at 150, 157.

50. Kingsley, "Third Sermon," 158–9.

51. [Charles Kingsley], "Mansfield's Paraguay, Brazil, and the Plate," *Frasers Magazine*, 54 (1856), 591–601, at 594–600; Kingsley, "The Locust-Swarms," in *The Good News of God: Sermons* (London, 1890), 161–8, at 163.

52. *The Letters of SGO: A Series of Letters on Public Affairs Written by the Rev. Lord Sidney Godolphin Osborne and Published in "The Times" 1844–1888*, ed. Arnold White (2 vol., London, n.d.), I, x, 189–90.

53. *The Letters of SGO*, I, 191–4, 216–20.

54. Martin Melosi, *The Sanitary City: Urban Infrastructure in America from Colonial Times to the Present* (Baltimore, 1999).

Chapter 3

1. Henry Wentworth Acland, *Memoir on the Cholera at Oxford, in the Year 1854, with Considerations Suggested by the Epidemic* (London, 1856), 6; Roderick McGrew, *Russia and the Cholera 1823–1832* (Madison, 1965), 128.

2. Acland, *Oxford*, 105.

3. Acland, *Oxford*, 106, 143.

4. Frances Kingsley, *Charles Kingsley* (2 vols, London, 1894), i. 65–6.

5. Acland, *Oxford*, 6.

6. Acland, *Oxford*, 6.

7. McGrew, *Russia*, 99, 127–9.

8. R. Nelson, *Asiatic Cholera: Its Origin and Spread in Asia, Africa, and Europe, Introduction into America through Canada; Remote and Proximate Causes, Symptoms and Pathology, and the Various Modes of Treatment Analyzed* (New York, 1866), 22.

9. E. O. Shakespeare, *Report on the Cholera in Europe and India* (Washington, 1890), 155.

10. Baldwin, *Contagion and the State*, 71.

11. *Cholera Bulletin* [New York], Aug. 8 1832, 116–17.

12. Albanesi, in Shakespeare, *Report on the Cholera in Europe and India*, 138.

13. Albanesi, in Shakespeare, *Report on the Cholera in Europe and India*, 136–7.

14. Ricardo Antonio Esteve, in Shakespeare, *Report on the Cholera in Europe and India*, 182.

15. Acland, *Oxford*, 105.

16. Acland, *Oxford*, 6–7.

17. Shakespeare, *Report on the Cholera in Europe and India*, 86.

18. Mary Douglas, *Purity and Danger: An Analysis of the Concepts of Pollution and Taboo* (London, 1966).

19. W. G. Lumley, *The Act for the More Speedy Removal of Nuisances, and the Prevention of Contagious Diseases, 9 & 10 Vic. c. 96* (London, 1846), 11, 13.

20. Michael Sigsworth, "Cholera in the Large Towns of the West and East Ridings, 1848–1893," PhD dissertation (Sheffield, 1991), 333.

21. Acland, *Oxford*, 99, 143.

22. Acland, *Oxford*, 90–2, 98–9.

23. Acland, *Oxford*, 96, 100, 105.

24. Nelson, *Asiastic Cholera*, 24, emphasis in original.

25. Michael Roth, "The Western Cholera Trail", 216, 221.

26. Acland, *Oxford*, 96–9; Rosenberg, *The Cholera Years*, 27, 86, 91.

27. A *Bradford Guardian*, quoted in Sigsworth, "Cholera," 149.

28. Alfred Stillé, *Cholera: Its Origin, History, Causation, Symptoms, Lesions, Prevention, and Treatment* (Philadelphia: Lea Brothers, 1885), 112–13.

29. Nelson, *Asiatic Cholera*, 74, 80.

30. *Cholera Bulletin*, 12, Aug. 1 1832, 91.

31. Shakespeare, *Report on the Cholera in Europe and India*, 3.

32. Acland, *Oxford*, 162.

33. Shakespeare, *Report on the Cholera in Europe and India*, 22.

34. Shakespeare, *Report on the Cholera in Europe and India*, 87–90.

35. Shakespeare, *Report on the Cholera in Europe and India*, 111.

36. Stillé, *Cholera*, 133–5; Nelson, *Asiatic Cholera*, 169, 193.

37. Shakespeare, *Report on the Cholera in Europe and India*, 50, 64.

38. Shakespeare, *Report on the Cholera in Europe and India*, 90.

39. Shakespeare, *Report on the Cholera in Europe and India*, 344, 866–7.

40. Roth, "Cholera Trail", 240, 391–2.

41. Shakespeare, *Report on the Cholera in Europe and India*, 208.

42. Quoted in Shakespeare, *Report on the Cholera in Europe and India*, 353–4.

43. N. Howard-Jones, "The Scientific Background of the International Sanitary Conferences, 1851–1938, 5," *WHO Chronicle*, 28 (1974), 455–70, at 458.

44. Baldwin, *Contagion*, 149–50, 172; Shakespeare, *Report on the Cholera in Europe and India*, 339; Stillé, *Cholera*, 117–21.

45. Stillé, *Cholera*, 120.

46. In Shakespeare, *Report on the Cholera in Europe and India*, 130.

47. Shakespeare, *Report on the Cholera in Europe and India*, 51.

48. Shakespeare, *Report on the Cholera in Europe and India*, 369.

49. Quoted in Baldwin, *Contagion*, 194–5, 212, 229–36.

50. Shakespeare, *Report on the Cholera in Europe and India*, 22–43, 368.

51. Shakespeare, *Report on the Cholera in Europe and India*, 4–5.

52. Quoted in Shakespeare, *Report on the Cholera in Europe and India*, 347, emphasis added.

53. N. Howard-Jones, "The Scientific Background of the International Sanitary Conferences, 1851–1938, 6," *WHO Chronicle*, 28 (1974), 495–508, at 497–502.

Chapter 4

1. Frank Snowden, *Naples in the Time of Cholera, 1884–1911* (Cambridge, 1995), 226.

2. The Analytical Sanitary Commission, "Records of the Results of Microscopical and Chemical Analyses of the Solids and Fluids consumed by all Classes of the Public," *Lancet*, Feb. 22, 1851, 216–25.

3. Reginald Orton, *An Essay on the Epidemic Cholera of India* (2nd edn, London, 1831), 287–8.

4. N. Howard-Jones, "The Scientific Background of the International Sanitary Conferences, 1851–1938. 2", *WHO Chronicle*, 28 (1974), 229–47, at 232.

5. John Austin, *Cholera Morbus: A Short and Faithful Account of the History, Progress, Causes, Symptoms, and Treatment of the Indian and Russian Cholera, Taken from Authentic Sources, with Cases as Related by Practitioners in India* (London, 1831), 6.

6. Whitelaw Ainslie, *Observations on the Cholera Morbus of India: A Letter Addressed to the Honourable Court of Directors of the East-India Company* (London, 1825), 3–5.

7. Hardin Weatherford, *A Treatise on Cholera, with the Causes, Symptoms, Mode of Prevention and Cure, on a New and Successful Plan* (Louisville, 1833), 36, 40, 44.

8. R. Nelson, *Asiatic Cholera: Its Origin and Spread in Asia, Africa, and Europe, Introduction into America through Canada; Remote and Proximate Causes, Symptoms and Pathology, and the Various Modes of Treatment Analyzed* (New York, 1866), iv, 28, 32–3, 36, 38–9, 56–8, 167–93.

9. E. A. Parkes, "Dr Snow on the Communication of Cholera," *British and Foreign Medico-Chirurgical Review*, 15 (1855), 449–63, at 463.

10. Parkes, "Dr Snow," 458.

11. Parkes, "Dr Snow," 458.

12. Richard Feachum, "Environmental Aspects of Cholera Epidemiology: III Transmission and Control," *Tropical Diseases Bulletin*, 79 (1982), 1–47.

13. William Farr, "Influence of Elevation on the Fatality of Cholera," *Journal of the Statistical Society of London*, 15 (1852), 155–83, 156–64; August Hirsch, *Handbook of Historical and Geographical Pathology. Vol. 1. Acute Infective Diseases* (London, 1883), 441–6.

14. Henry Wentworth Acland, *Memoir on the Cholera at Oxford, in the Year 1854, with Considerations Suggested by the Epidemic* (London, 1856), 14–20, 50–2.

15. Alexander Wynter Blyth, *A Dictionary of Hygiene and Public Health* (London 1876), s.v., "Putrefaction."

16. John Snow, "On Continuous Molecular Changes, More Particularly in their Relation to Epidemic Diseases," in *Snow on Cholera—A Reprint of Two Papers by John Snow, MD*, together with a Biographical Memoir by B. W. Richardson, MD, and an Introduction by Wade Hampton Frost (New York, 1936).

17. Hirsch, *Handbook*, 476, 492–3.

18. H. W. Bellew, *The History of Cholera in India from 1862 to 1881: Being a Descriptive and Statistical Account of the Disease Derived from the Published Official Reports of the Several Provincial Governments during*

that *Period and Mainly in Illustration of the Relation between Cholera Activity and Climatic Conditions together with Original Observations on the Causes and Nature of Cholera* (London, 1885), v, 5.

19. Bellew, *History of Cholera*, 5–12.

20. Parkes, "Dr Snow," 463.

21. Sheldon Watts, *Epidemics and History: Disease, Power and Imperialism* (New Haven, 1997), 168.

22. Walter Vought, *A Chapter on Cholera for Lay Readers* (Philadelphia 1893), 10.

23. Richard J. Evans, *Death in Hamburg: Society and Politics in the Cholera Years 1830–1910* (London, 1990), 268.

Chapter 5

1. Robert Koch, "An Address on Cholera and its Bacillus," trans. W. Watson-Cheyne, in E. O. Shakespeare, *Report on the Cholera in Europe and India* (Washington, 1890), 450.

2. William Summers, "Cholera and Plague in India: The Bacteriophage Inquiry of 1927–1936," *Journal of the History of Medicine and Allied Sciences*, 48 (1993), 275–301.

3. Robert Koch, "Further Researches on Cholera," *British Medical Journal*, 2 & 9 Jan. 1886, 6–8, 62–6, at 7.

4. Leonard Rogers, *Cholera and its Treatment* (London, 1911), 54.

5. Koch, "Further Researches," 7.

6. Robert Koch, "An Address on Cholera and its Bacillus," *British Medical Journal*, Aug. 30 and Sept. 6 1884, 403–7, 453–9, at 403.

7. "Dr Koch's Newly Described Cholera-Organism," *British Medical Journal*, Oct. 27, 1883, 828–9, at 828.

8. Robert Koch, "Third Report of the German Cholera Commission," quoted in N. Howard-Jones, "The Scientific Background of the International Sanitary Conferences, 1851–1938, 3," *WHO Chronicle*, 28 (1974), 369–84, at 376.

9. Koch, "Address on Cholera and its Bacillus," in Shakespeare, *Report on the Cholera in Europe and India*, 453.

10. Koch, "Further Researches," 63–4.

11. Koch, "Address on Cholera and its Bacillus," in Shakespeare, *Report on the Cholera in Europe and India*, 465–7.

12. August Hirsch, *Handbook of Historical and Geographical Pathology. Vol. 1. Acute Infective Diseases* (London, 1883), 480–2.

13. E. E. Klein and Henege Gibbes, "British Cholera Commission," in Shakespeare, *Report on the Cholera in Europe and India*, 509–13.

14. Koch, "Address on Cholera and its Bacillus," in Shakespeare, *Report on the Cholera in Europe and India*, 455; cf Koch, "Further Researches," 64.

15. Koch, "Address on Cholera and its Bacillus," in Shakespeare, *Report on the Cholera in Europe and India*, 457.

16. Mariko Ogawa, "Uneasy Bedfellows: Science and Politics in the Refutation of Koch's Bacterial Theory of Cholera," *Bulletin of the History of Medicine*, 74 (2000), 671–707.

17. Koch, "Further Researches," 6–7.

18. Hirsch, *Handbook*, 477–9.

19. Koch, "Further Researches," 64.

20. E. E. Klein, *The Bacteria in Asiatic Cholera* (New York, 1889), 122; Klein and Gibbes, "British Cholera Commission," in Shakespeare, *Report on the Cholera in Europe and India*, 498–503.

21. Klein and Gibbes, "British Cholera Commission," in Shakespeare, *Report on the Cholera in Europe and India*, 480–1, 507, 513–15.

22. W. E van Heyningen and John R. Seal, *Cholera: The American Scientific Experience, 1947–1980* (Boulder, CO, 1983), 32.

23. Klein and Gibbes, "British Cholera Commission," in Shakespeare, *Report on the Cholera in Europe and India*, 512.

24. Robert Koch, *Professor Koch on the Bacteriological Diagnosis of Cholera, Water-Filtration and Cholera, and the Cholera in German during the Winter of 1892–93*, trans. George Duncan (New York, 1895), 28.

25. Shakespeare, *Report on the Cholera in Europe and India*, 711, 818.

26. Shakespeare, *Report on the Cholera in Europe and India*, 713–14.

27. R. Nelson, *Asiatic Cholera: Its Origin and Spread in Asia, Africa, and Europe, Introduction into America through Canada; Remote and Proximate Causes, Symptoms and Pathology, and the Various Modes of Treatment Analyzed* (New York, 1866), 187.

28. Michael Durey, *The Return of the Plague* (Dublin, 1979), 126.

29. Van Heyningen and Seal, *Cholera*, 50.

30. M. M. Levine and J. B. Kaper, "Cholera Pathogenesis and Vaccine Development," in B. S. Drasar and B. D. Forrest, *Cholera and the Ecology of* Vibrio cholerae (London, 1996), 125–86, at 141–2.

31. Melissa R. Kaufman and Ronald K. Taylor, "The Toxin-Coregulated Pilus: Biogenesis and Function," in I. Kaye Wachsmuth, Paul A. Blake, and Ørjan Olsvik (eds), *Vibrio Cholerae and Cholera: Molecular to Global Perspectives* (Washington, 1994), 187–202, at 187.

32. Eric S. Krukonis and Victor J. DiRita, "From Motility to Virulence: Sensing and Responding to Environmental Signals in *Vibrio Cholerae*," *Current Opinion in Microbiology*, 6 (2003), 186–90, at 187.

33. Matthew K. Waldor and John Mekalanos, "Lysogenic Conversion by a Filamentous Phage Encoding Cholera Toxin," *Science*, 272/5270 (1996), 1910–14.

34. Joachim Reidl and Karl Klose, "*Vibrio Cholerae* and Cholera: Out of the Water and into the Host," *FEMS Microbiology Reviews*, 26 (2002), 125–39, at 133.

35. Reidl and Klose, "*Vibrio Cholerae* and Cholera," 134.

Chapter 6

1. A. J. H. Russell, *A Memorandum on the Epidemiology of Cholera* (Geneva, 1925), 40.

2. Dhiman Barua, "History of Cholera," in Dhiman Barua and William B. Greenough III (eds), *Cholera* (New York, 1992), 1–36, at 5.

3. Dhiman Barua and Michael Merson, "Prevention and Control of Cholera," in Barua and Greenough (eds), *Cholera*, 329–49, at 336.

4. J. Glenn Morris Jr, "Non-O1 Group 1 *Vibrio cholerae* Strains not Associated with Epidemic Disease," in Kaye Wachsmuth, Paul A. Blake, and Ørjan Olsvik (eds), *Vibrio Cholerae and Cholera: Molecular to Global Perspectives*, (Washington, 1994), 103–15, at 103–9.

5. Paul Blake, "Endemic Cholera in Australia and the United States," in Wachsmuth et al. (eds), *Vibrio cholerae*, 309–19, at, 311, 313.

6. Kathryn Cottingham, Deborah Chiavelli, and Ronald K. Taylor, "Environmental Microbe and Human Pathogen: The Ecology and Microbiology of *Vibrio Cholerae*," *Frontiers in Ecology and Environment*, 1 (2003), 80–6, at 80.

7. Erin K. Lipp, Anwar Huq, and Rita R. Colwell, "Effects of Global Climate on Infectious Disease: The Cholera Model," *Clinical Microbiology Reviews*, 15 (2002), 757–70, at 759.

8. Rita Colwell and William Spira, "Ecology," in Barua and Greenough (eds), *Cholera*, 107–27.

9. Roger Glass and Robert Black, "The Epidemiology of Cholera," in Barua and Greenough (eds), *Cholera*, 129–50, at 130, 138.

10. Stephen Richardson, "Animal Models," in Wachsmuth et al. (eds), *Vibrio cholerae*, 203–26, at 212.

11. Stephen Richardson, "Host Susceptibility," in Wachsmuth et al. (eds), *Vibrio cholerae*, 273–89, at 280.

12. Tanja Popovic et al., "Detection of Cholera Toxin Genes," in Wachsmuth et al. (eds), *Vibrio cholerae*, 41–52, at 41.

13. Rita Colwell and Anwar Huq, "Vibrios in the Environment," in Wachsmuth et al. (eds), *Vibrio cholerae*, 117–33, at 121, 129–30.

14. W. E. van Heyningen and John R. Seal, *Cholera: The American Scientific Experience, 1947–1980* (Boulder, CO, 1983), 249–50.

15. D. Mahalanabis et al., "Clinical Management of Cholera," in Barua and Greenough (eds), *Cholera*, 253–83, at 270–2.

16. http://www.emro.who.int/sudan/media/pdf/Cholera CaseDefinition.pdf, accessed Aug. 9 2008.

17. Claudio Lanata and Walter Mendoza, *Improving Diarrhoea Estimates* (Geneva, 2002); http://www.who.int/child adolescent health/ documents/pdfs/improving diarrhoea estimates.pdf, accessed Aug. 9 2008, 4.

18. J. Clemens et al., "Public Health Considerations for the Use of Cholera Vaccines," in Wachsmuth et al. (eds), *Vibrio cholerae*, 425–40, at 431; van Heyningen and Seal, *Cholera*, 245.

19. Barua and Merson, "Prevention and Control of Cholera," 340; Clemens et al., "Public Health Considerations for the Use of Cholera Vaccines," 431, 435.

20. Jan Holmgren et al., "Protective Oral Cholera Vaccine," in Wachsmuth et al. (eds), *Vibrio cholerae*, 415–24, at 422.

21. Shahjahan Kabir, "Cholera Vaccines: The Current Status and Problems," *Reviews in Medical Microbiology*, 16 (2005), 101–16, at 111–12.

22. Barua and Merson, "Prevention and Control of Cholera," 347, emphasis in original.

23. Robert Tauxe et al., "The Latin American Epidemic," in Wachsmuth et al. (eds), *Vibrio cholerae*, 321–44, at 340.

24. Van Heyningen and Seal, *cholerae*, 212–13.

25. Eugene Gangarosa and Robert Tauxe, "Epilogue: The Latin American Cholera Epidemic," 351–8, at 358.

26. Robert Tauxe et al., "The Future of Cholera," in Wachsmuth et al. (eds), *Vibrio cholerae*, 443–53, at 443.

27. Gangarosa and Tauxe, "Epilogue," 358; Tauxe et al., "The Future of Cholera," 452.

28. Thandavarayan Ramamurthy, Shinji Yamasaki, Yoshifumi Takeda, and G. B. Nair, "*Vibrio cholerae* O139 Bengal: Odyssey of a Fortuitous Variant," *Microbes and Infection*, 5 (2003), 329–44 at 331.

29. Robert Tauxe et al., "Latin American Epidemic," 334–6.

30. Tauxe et al., "Latin American Epidemic," 341.

31. Gangarosa and Tauxe, "Epilogue," 353–4, emphasis in original.

32. Tauxe et al., "Latin American Epidemic," 334.

33. Michael L. Bennish, "Cholera: Pathophysiology, Clinical Features, and Treatment," in Wachsmuth et al. (eds), *Vibrio cholerae*, 229–55, at 230.

34. Barua and Merson, "Prevention and Control of Cholera," 333.

35. Barua and Merson, "Prevention and Control of Cholera," 337, 340.

36. Barua and Merson, "Prevention and Control of Cholera," 343.

37. Andrew Collins, "Vulerability to Coastal Cholera Ecology," *Social Science and Medicine*, 57 (2003), 1397–1407, at 1398.

38. Tauxe et al., "The Latin American Epidemic," 342.

FURTHER READING

The literature on cholera is enormous but compartment-alized. I draw here on three bodies of work: cholera histories, nineteenth-century accounts, and modern cholera science.

1. Cholera histories

Cholera history began in the late 1950s as social historians appreciated its centrality for nineteenth-century Europe. Important programmatic works were Louis Chevalier (ed.), *Le Choléra: La Première Épidémie du XIXe Siècle* (La Roche-sur-Yon, 1958); Roderick McGrew, "The First Cholera Epidemic and Social History," *Bulletin of the History of Medicine*, 34 (1960), 61–73; Asa Briggs, "Cholera and Society," *Past and Present*, 119 (1961), 76–96; Charles Rosenberg, "Cholera in Nineteenth Century Europe: A Tool for Social and Economic Analysis," *Comparative Studies in Society and History*, 8 (1966), 452–63. By the 1960s cholera was the most popular historical disease. For the United States these themes were reflected in Rosenberg's *The Cholera Years: The United States in 1832, 1849, and 1866* (Chicago, 1962), more cultural history than history of an epidemic. For Europe, Roderick McGrew's *Russia and the Cholera 1823–1832* (Madison, 1965) and Norman Longmate's semi-popular *King Cholera* (London, 1966) set out dramatic themes that still shape scholarship. Some of these (like cholera riots) were enlarged in Michael Durey's careful *The Return of the Plague* (Dublin, 1979), which dealt with England's response to 1832. Exemplary works for France are Patrice Bourdelais and Jean-Yves Raulot, *Une Peur Bleue: Histoire du Choléra en France, 1832–1854* (Paris, 1987), and, for Germany, Olaf Briese's four-volume *Angst in den Zeiten der Cholera* (Berlin, 2003). The latter volumes are an impressive record of responses to cholera—in letters and in poetry. The persistence of interest in cholera among scholars of Victorian culture and literature is evident in Pamela Gilbert, *Cholera and Nation: Doctoring the Social Body in Victorian England* (Albany, NY, 2008). *Visages du Choléra* by Patrice Bourdelais and André Dodin (Paris, 1987) is a wonderful collection of cholera illustrations.

By 1985, cholera histories had shifted to local studies. To the exemplary works by François Delaporte (*Disease and Civilisation, the Cholera in Paris, 1832*, trans. A. Goldhammer (Cambridge, MA: 1986)), Richard Evans (*Death in Hamburg: Society and Politics in the Cholera Years 1830–1910* (London, 1990)), and Frank Snowden (*Naples in the Time of Cholera, 1884–1911* (Cambridge, 1995)) can be added the doctoral dissertations of Gerald Kearns ("Aspects of Cholera, Society, and Space in Nineteenth Century England and Wales" (Cambridge, 1985)); Michael Sigsworth ("Cholera in the Large Towns of the West and East Ridings, 1848–1893" (Sheffield Polytechnic, 1991)), and Michael Roth, "The Western Cholera Trail: Studies in the Urban Response to Epidemic Disease in the Trans-Mississippi West, 1848–1850" (Santa Barbara, 1993)). There are many other article- and book-length local studies. A short, hard-hitting exemplar is Frank Snowden, "Cholera in Barletta, 1910," *Past and Present*, 132 (1991), 67–103.

By the 1990s cholera history had expanded to colonial and post-colonial contexts. Indian cholera had been treated by Ira Klein in "Cholera: Theory and Treatment in Nineteenth Century India," *Journal of Indian History* (1980), 35–51, and in "Imperialism,

Ecology, and Disease," *Indian Economic and Social History Journal*, 31/4 (1994), 491–518, and in broader context in the work of David Arnold and Mark Harrison—by Arnold in "Cholera and Colonialism in British India," *Past and Present*, 113 (1986), 118–51, and *Colonizing the Body: State Medicine and Epidemic Disease in Nineteenth-Century India* (Berkeley and Los Angeles, 1993), and by Harrison in *Public Health in British India: Anglo-Indian Preventive Medicine 1859–1914* (Cambridge, 1994), *Climates and Constitutions: Health, Race, Environment and British Imperialism in India 1600–1850* (New Delhi, 1999), and "A Question of Locality: The Identity of Cholera in British India, 1860–1890," in David Arnold (ed.), *Warm Climates and Western Medicine: The Emergence of Tropical Medicine* (Amsterdam, 1996), 133–59. Cholera often figured in works on nineteenth-century cultural confrontation on health matters, as, for China, in Kerrie MacPherson, *A Wilderness of Marshes: The Origins of Public Health in Shanghai, 1843–1893* (Hong Kong, 1987) and Ruth Rogaski, *Hygienic Modernity: Meanings of Health and Disease in Treaty-Port China* (Berkeley and Los Angeles, 2004). In "Excremental Colonialism: Public Health and the Poetics of Pollution," *Critical Inquiry*, 21 (1995), 640–69, and later *Colonial Pathologies: American Tropical Medicine, Race, and Hygiene in the Philippines* (Durham, NC, 2006), Warwick Anderson laid out a more critical perspective for colonializing cholera, and broadened the frame geographically. Not surprisingly, a theme of bitterness, characteristic of much post-colonial scholarship, finds ample scope in the persistence of preventable cholera, e.g., Vijay Prashad, "Native Dirt/Imperial Ordure: The Cholera of 1832 and the Morbid Resolutions of Modernity," *Journal of Historical Sociology* (1994), 243–60; Sheldon Watts, *Epidemics and History: Disease, Power and Imperialism* (New Haven, 1997); and "From Rapid Change to Stasis: Official Responses to Cholera in British-Ruled India: 1860–c. 1921," *Journal of World History*, 12 (2001), 321–74. Many of these themes—local studies, colonial (and racial) attitudes are combined in Charles Briggs and Clara Mantini-Briggs, *Stories in the Time of Cholera: Racial Profiling during a Medical Nightmare* (Berkeley and Los Angeles, 2003), focusing on a remote area of north-eastern Venezuela.

These works were social histories primarily; another strain of work took up theory and practice with regard to prevention, and, separately, therapy. With respect to the former, many works saw cholera as the site of the grand battle between old and new, error and truth, anticontagionism and contagionism (ultimately matured in germ theory and bacteriology). Erwin Ackerknecht's classic stating of the issues in "Anticontagionism between 1821 and 1867," *Bulletin of the History of Medicine*, 22 (1948), 562–93, was put to exhaustive test in Peter Baldwin, *Contagion and the State in Europe, 1830–1930* (New York, 1999), which included two massive chapters on cholera. Earlier Margaret Pelling (*Cholera, Fever, and English Medicine, 1825–1865* (Oxford, 1978)) and John Eyler (*Victorian Social Medicine: The Ideas and Methods of William Farr* (Baltimore, 1979)) had challenged the usual dichotomies by making clear the centrality of contingent contagionism and zymotic theory.

Cholera has been the occasion of myth-making, notes Norman Howard-Jones ("Choleranomalies: The Unhistory of Medicine as Exemplified by Cholera," *Perspectives in Biology and Medicine*, 15 (1972), 422–33). There has remained great interest in the story of John Snow. The current standard biography, *Cholera, Chloroform, and the Science of Medicine: A Life of John Snow* (Oxford, 2003), a work long in preparation by an interdisciplinary group (Peter Vinten-Johansen, Howard Brody, Nigel Paneth, Stephen Rachman, and Michael Rip), is illuminating with regard to Snow's creativity and methods, but fails adequately to contextualize. The best access to Snow's seminal works (though not to his important periodical publications) remains *Snow on Cholera: A Reprint of Two Papers by John Snow, MD, together with a Biographical Memoir by B. W. Richardson MD, and an Introduction by Wade Hampton Frost* (New York, 1936). This includes both the 2nd (1855) edition of "On the Mode of Communication of Cholera" and "On Continuous Molecular Changes, More Particularly in their Relation to Epidemic Diseases" (1853). Snow's emergence as a mythic figure is explored in Jan Vandenbroucke, H. M. Beukers, and H. Eelkman Rooda, "Who Made John Snow a Hero?" *American Journal of Epidemiology*, 133 (1991), 967–73; and Kari S. McLeod, "Our Sense of Snow: The Myth of John Snow in Medical Geography," *Social Science and Medicine*, 50 (2000), 923–35. But see also George Davey-Smith, "Behind the Broad Street Pump: Aetiology, Epidemiology and Prevention of Cholera in 19th-Century Britain," *International Journal of Epidemiology*, 31 (2002), 920–32, and Thomas Koch and Kenneth Denike, "Rethinking John Snow's South London Study: A Bayesian Evaluation and Recalculation", *Social Science and Medicine*, 63 (2006), 271–83. Issues of water and disease during the Snow years and after have been explored by Bill Luckin (*Pollution and Control: A Social History of the Thames in the Nineteenth Century* (Bristol, 1986)) and Christopher Hamlin (*A Science of Impurity: Water Analysis in Nineteenth-Century Britain* (Bristol, and Berkeley and Los Angeles, 1990)).

The cholera work of other theorists, including Koch, but also Pettenkofer, has received less concentrated attention. Koch's methodological revolution has been carefully examined by K. Codell Carter, "Koch's Postulates in relation to the Work of Jacob Henle and Edwin Klebs," *Medical History*, 29 (1985), 353–74, and William Coleman, "Koch's Comma Bacillus: The First Year," *Bulletin of the History of Medicine*, 61 (1987), 315–42.

Mariko Ogawa, "Uneasy Bedfellows: Science and Politics in the Refutation of Koch's Bacterial Theory of Cholera," *Bulletin of the History of Medicine*, 74 (2000), 671–707, examines British antagonism to Koch, while Michael Worboys, *Spreading Germs: Disease Theories and Medical Practice in Britain, 1865–1900* (Cambridge, 2000), sets the context. A fine study of an underappreciated Indian theorist is Jeremy Isaacs, "D. D. Cunningham and the Aetiology of Cholera in British India, 1869–1897," *Medical History*, 42 (1998), 279–305. The ambiguous role of science in the international response to cholera was well handled in six articles by Norman Howard-Jones, "The Scientific Background of the International Sanitary Conferences, 1851–1938," *WHO Chronicle*, 28 (1974), 159–71, 229–47, 369–84, 414–26, 455–70, 495–508. The subject deserves more attention.

Cholera therapy has usually been the focus of ridicule. The exemplar is Norman Howard-Jones, "Cholera Therapy in the Nineteenth Century," *Journal of the History of Medicine*, 27 (1972), 372–95. Cross-cultural issues are thoughtfully addressed in Dhrub Kumar Singh, "Cholera in Two Contrasting Pathies in Nineteenth Century India," *Disquisitions on the Past and Present*, 13 (Oct. 2005), 103–26. Vaccination has generally received a more balanced and insightful treatment. Helpful are Charles Cameron, "Anti-Cholera Inoculation," *Nineteenth Century*, 8 (1885), 338–52; George H. Bornside, "Jaime Ferran and Preventive Inoculation against Cholera," *Bulletin of the History of Medicine*, 55 (1981), 516–32, and "Waldemar Haffkine's Cholera Vaccines and the Ferran–Haffkine Priority Dispute," *Journal of the History of Medicine*, 37/4 (1982), 399–422; I. Löwy, "From Guinea Pigs to Man: The Development of Haffkine's Anticholera Vaccine," *Journal of the History of Medicine*, 47 (1992), 270–309, and especially William Summers, "Cholera and Plague in India: The Bacteriophage

Inquiry of 1927–1936," *Journal of the History of Medicine and Allied Sciences*, 48 (1993), 275–301. Haffkine's own reflections (*Protective Inoculation against Cholera* (Calcutta, 1913)) are also intriguing, as are Leonard Rogers's on the emergence of rehydration in *Cholera and its Treatment* (London, 1911) and *Happy Toil: Fifty-Five Years of Tropical Medicine* (London, 1950).

Few historians have ventured into post-Kochian cholera science during the golden age of bacteriology. To the practitioner–historians W. E. van Heyningen and John R. Seal (*Cholera: The American Scientific Experience, 1947–1980* (Boulder, CO, 1983)), it was an era of equivocal work based on erroneous assumptions about toxic action, but that overstates. That work was carefully and lovingly chronicled by R. Pollitzer in the early 1950s, a masterwork of scientific reviewing. The monograph (*Cholera* (Geneva, 1958)) is rare, but the work is accessible as a series of "Cholera Studies" in the *Bulletin of the World Health Organization*, 10 (1954), 421–61; 12 (1955), 311–58, 777–875, 944–1007, 1075–1199; 13 (1955), 1–25; 16 (1957), 67–162, 123–99, 295–430, 783–857. (In a few cases Pollitzer was aided by co-authors.)

2. Nineteenth-century accounts

What "cholera" meant to Europeans before the nineteenth century is considered in George Rousseau and David Boyd Haycock, "Coleridge's Choleras: Cholera Morbus, Asiatic Cholera, and Dysentery in Early Nineteenth-Century England," *Bulletin of the History of Medicine*, 77 (2003), 298–31. The term is encountered in texts, treatises, and medical dictionaries. I have relied mainly on Robert James's *Medicinal Dictionary* (3 vols, London, 1743–5). For a sense of cholera's incidence, see John Heysham, *Observations on the Bills of Mortality, in Carlisle, for the year MDCCLXXXIII* (Carlisle,

1784); and for its routine character, Charles Frankland, *Travels to and from Constantinopole in the years 1827 and 1828* (2 vols, London, 1829).

Nineteenth-century cholera treatises abound. I have sought to include a variety of genres, productions of the moment as well as of a lifetime, and to represent a range of perspectives. I have relied heavily on a few relatively obscure authors: the Oxford professor of medicine W. H. Acland (1815–1900), the Canadian physician-revolutionary Robert Nelson (1794–1873), the Anglo-Indian surgeons Reginald Orton (1790–1835), N. Charles Macnamara (1832–1918), and John McPherson (1817–90), the French medical polymath Raoul-Henri-Joseph Scoutetten (1799–1871), the Philadelphia society physician Alfred Stillé (1813–1900), and the American pathologist E. O. Shakespeare (1846–1900). Their biographies are available in standard medical or biographical dictionaries.

Others may be divided by period. Important works on the early cholera in India are Whitelaw Ainslie, *Observations on the Cholera Morbus of India: A Letter Address to the Honourable Court of Directors of the East-India Company* (London, 1825), James Annesley, *Sketches of the Most Prominent Diseases of India… Statistical and Topographical Reports of the Diseases of the Different Divisions of the Army under the Madras Presidency….* (2nd edn, London, 1829), James Kennedy, *The History of the Contagious Cholera* (2nd edn, London, 1832), and Orton's *An Essay on the Epidemic Cholera of India* (2nd edn, London, 1831).

Attempts to make sense of the new disease as it spread elsewhere in the first half of the nineteenth century are evident in *Papers Relative to the Disease Now Called Cholera Spasmodica in India; Now Prevailing in the North of Europe* (London, 1831); *Rapport sur le Choléra Morbus, lu a L'Académie de Médecine, en Séance Générale, les 26 et*

30 Juillet 1831 (Paris, 1831), *Report of the Committee of Internal Health on the Asiatic Cholera, together with a Report of the City Physician on the Cholera Hospital* (Boston, 1849), John Austin, *Cholera Morbus: A Short and Faithful Account of the History, Progress, Causes, Symptoms, and Treatment of the Indian and Russian Cholera* (London, 1831); F. J. V. Broussais, *Le Choléra-Morbus Épidémique, Observé et Traité selon la Méthode Physiologique* (Paris, 1832), F. Bisset Hawkins, *History of the Spasmodic Cholera of Russia; Including a Copious Account of the Disease which has Prevailed in India, and which has Travelled, under that Name, from Asia into Europe* (London, 1831), Hardin Weatherford, *A Treatise on Cholera, with the Causes, Symptoms, Mode of Prevention and Cure, on a New and Successful Plan* (Louisville, 1833); R. H. Scoutetten, *A Medical and Topographical History of the Cholera Morbus, Including the Mode of Prevention and Treatment*, trans. A. Sidney Doane (Boston, 1832), and Thomas Shapter, *The History of the Cholera in Exeter in 1832* (London, 1849). *The Cholera Bulletin*, an 1832 New York periodical, has been reprinted with introduction by Charles Rosenberg (New York, 1972).

Important works for later in the century are E. A. Parkes, "Dr Snow on the Communication of Cholera," *British and Foreign Medico-Chirurgical Review*, 15 (1855), 449–63, Acland's *Memoir on the Cholera at Oxford in the year 1854* (London, 1856), Nelson's *Asiatic Cholera: Its Origin and Spread in Asia, Africa, and Europe...Remote and Proximate Causes, Symptoms and Pathology, and the Various Modes of Treatment Analysed* (New York, 1866), James Christie, *Cholera Epidemics in East Africa* (London, 1876), John Murray, *Observations on the Pathology and Treatment of Cholera* (New York, 1874), Alfred Stillé, *Cholera: Its Origin, History, Causation, Symptoms, Lesions, Prevention, and Treatment* (Philadelphia, 1885), H. W. Bellew, *The History of Cholera in India from 1862 to 1881: Being a Descriptive and Statistical Account of the Disease Derived from the Published Official Reports...Mainly in Illustration of the Relation between Cholera Activity and Climatic Conditions* (London, 1885), August Hirsch, *Handbook of Historical and Geographical Pathology. Vol. 1. Acute Infective Diseases,* trans. Charles Creighton (London, 1883), Walter Vought, *A Chapter on Cholera for Lay Readers* (Philadelphia, 1893), Joseph Fayrer, *The Natural History and Epidemiology of Cholera* (London, 1888), and Cassim Izzeddine, *Organisation et Réformes Sanitaires au Hedjaz et le* Pélerinage *de 1329 (1911–12)* (Constantinople, 1913).

For the mid 1880s, the age of Koch, the great source is Shakespeare's *Report on the Cholera in Europe and India* (Washington, 1890). It includes Koch's major papers, as well as a motley group of other reports and Shakespeare's candid assessments of them. Others of Koch's papers, in slightly different translation, are in the *British Medical Journal* (1883–6). Klein's critique is in *The Bacteria in Asiatic Cholera* (New York, 1889), while Koch's views on Hamburg and water are collected in *Professor Koch on the Bacteriological Diagnosis of Cholera, Water-Filtration and Cholera, and the Cholera in Germany during the Winter of 1892–93,* trans. George Duncan (New York, 1895).

Non-medical works are also important. The best cholera novel is Charles Kingsley, *Two Years Ago.* My citations are from *The Works of Charles Kingsley,* (Philadelphia, 1899). The views of Kingsley's fellow reformer Osborne are collected in *The Letters of SGO: A Series of Letters on Public Affairs Written by the Rev. Lord Sidney Godolphin Osborne and Published in 'The Times' 1844–1888,* ed. Arnold White (2 vols, London, n.d.), and of my ancestor Cyrus Hamlin in *Among the Turks* (New York, 1877).

Late-nineteenth-century writers also took up the question of cholera's prehistory in India. Among the most important works were James Bontius, *An Account of the Diseases, Natural History,* and Medicines, of the East Indies (London, 1769), R. H. Scoutetten, *Histoire Chronologique Topographique et Étymologique du Choléra depuis la Haute Antiquité jusqu'a son Invasion en France en 1832* (Paris, 1869), Macpherson's *Annals of Cholera from the Earliest Period to the Year 1817* (London, 1872; 2nd edn, 1884), Macnamara's *A History of Asiatic Cholera* (London, 1876), and J. Semmelink, *Geschiedenis der Cholera in Oost-Indië Vóór 1817* (Utrecht, 1885). The Germanic scholarship being brought to bear is evident in Julius Jolly, *Indian Medicine*, trans. with notes by C. G. Kashikar (3rd edn, New Delhi, 1994).

3. Modern cholera science

Modern cholera science merges into historical scholarship with regard to the question of cholera's antiquity. As to how and whether European cholera differed from the post-1817 cholera, the dominant modern view is N. Howard-Jones, "Cholera Nomenclature and Nosology: A Historical Note," *Bulletin of the World Health Organization*, 51 (1974), 317–24, or D. E. S. Stewart-Tull, "Vaba, Haiza, Kholera, Foklune or Cholera: In Any Language Still the Disease of Seven Pandemics," *Journal of Applied Microbiology*, 91 (2001), 580–91. A pioneer in the dissenting view was the renowned cholera pathologist S. N. De, in his *Cholera: Its Pathology and Pathogenesis* (Edinburgh, 1961), though see also A. J. H. Russell, *A Memorandum on the Epidemiology of Cholera* (Geneva, 1925). Insightful on the Ola Bibi question is Sunder Lal Hora, "Worship of the Deities Olā, Jholā, and Bōn Bibī in Lower Bengal," *Journal and Proceedings of the Asiatic Society of Bengal*, NS 29 (1933), 1–4.

The best access to post-Pollitzer cholera science is through the periodic compendia, compilations of the views of experts. Oscar Felsenfeld's *The Cholera Problem* (St Louis, 1967), was semi-popular, but the first of the compendia, *Cholera* (Philadelphia, 1974), edited by William Burrows and Dhiman Barua, was not. Three such volumes appeared in the 1990s, largely in response to the resurgence of cholera in the Americas. *Cholera* (New York, 1992), edited by Dhiman Barua and William B. Greenough III, was in many ways an update of the earlier work. *Vibrio Cholerae and Cholera: Molecular to Global Perspectives*, edited by I. Kaye Wachsmuth, Paul A. Blake, and Ørjan Olsvik, and published by the American Society for Microbiology, was comprehensive, but reflected the revolution in molecular genetics as well. Finally, *Cholera and the Ecology of Vibrio cholerae* (London, 1996), edited by B. S. Drasar and B. D. Forrest, reflected the re-emergence of interest in what *Vibrio cholerae* was doing outside human bodies, and the many ways environmental factors might exacerbate or mitigate its pathogenicity.

There have been profound changes in cholera science post 1996. For these (and for a few pre-1996 issues) I have relied on review articles and the occasional research report. Among the most important have been Andrew Collins, "Vulerability to Coastal Cholera Ecology," *Social Science and Medicine*, 57 (2003), 1397–1407 (and Collins's superb discussion of "The Geography of Cholera" in Drasar and Forrest (eds), *Cholera and the Ecology of Vibrio Cholerae*); Kathryn Cottingham, Deborah Chiavelli, and Ronald K. Taylor, "Environmental Microbe and Human Pathogen: The Ecology and Microbiology of *Vibrio Cholerae*," *Frontiers in Ecology and Environment*, 1 (2003), 80–6; B. S. Drasar, "Pathogenesis and Ecology: The Case of Cholera," *Journal of Tropical Medicine and Hygiene*, 95 (1992), 365–72; Richard Feachum, "Environmental Aspects of Cholera Epidemiology: III Transmission and Control," *Tropical Diseases Bulletin*, 79 (1982), 1–47; David C. Griffith, Louise Kelly-Hope, and Mark A. Miller, "Review of Reported Cholera Outbreaks

Worldwide, 1995–2005", *American Journal of Tropical Medicine and Hygiene*, 75 (2006), 973–7; Shahjahan Kabir, "Cholera Vaccines: The Current Status and Problems," *Reviews in Medical Microbiology*, 16 (2005), 101–16; Eric Krukonis and Victor J. DiRita, "From Motility to Virulence: Sensing and Responding to Environmental Signals in *Vibrio Cholerae*," *Current Opinion in Microbiology*, 6 (2003), 186–90; Erin K. Lipp, Anwar Huq, and Rita R. Colwell, "Effects of Global Climate on Infectious Disease: The Cholera Model," *Clinical Microbiology Reviews*, 15 (2002), 757–70; Mercedes Pascual, Menno J. Bouma, and Andrew P. Dobson, "Cholera and Climate: Revisiting the Quantitative Evidence," *Microbes and Infection*, 4 (2002), 237–45; Thandavarayan Ramamurthy, Shinji Yamasaki, Yoshifumi Takeda, and G. B. Nair, "*Vibrio Cholerae* O139 Bengal: Odyssey of a Fortuitous Variant," *Microbes and Infection*, 5 (2003), 329–44; Joachim Reidl and Karl Klose, "*Vibrio Cholerae* and Cholera: Out of the Water and into the Host," *FEMS Microbiology Reviews*, 26 (2002), 125–39; Johanna Santamaria and Gary Toranzos, "Enteric Pathogens and Soil: A Short Review," *International Microbiology*, 6 (2003), 5–9; Paul Shears, "Recent Developments in Cholera," *Current Opinion in Infectious Diseases*, 14 (2001), 553–8; G. Uma, M. Chandrasekaren, Yoshifumi Takeda, and G. Balakrish Nair, "Recent Advances in Cholera Genetics," *Current Science*, 85 (2003), 1538–45; Mathew K. Waldor and John Mekalanos, "Lysogenic Conversion by a Filamentous Phage Encoding Cholera Toxin," *Science*, 272/5270 (1996), 1910–14; Jane Zuckerman, Lars Rombo, and Alain Fisch, "The True Burden and Risk of Cholera: Implications for Prevention and Control," *Lancet Infectious Disease*, 7 (2007), 521–30. And, for comparison with other diarrheal disease, Umesh Parashar, Erik Hummelman, Joseph Bresee, Mark Miller, and Roger Glass, "Global Illness and Deaths Caused by Rotavirus Disease in Children," *Emerging Infectious Disease*, 9 (2003), 565–72.

INDEX